MEASURING FORENSIC PSYCHIATRIC AND MENTAL HEALTH NURSING INTERACTIONS

Measuring Forensic Psychiatric and Mental Health Nursing Interactions

DAVID ROBINSON
VAL REED

Avebury

Aldershot • Brookfield USA • Hong Kong • Singapore • Sydney

Published by
Avebury
Ashgate Publishing Limited
Gower House
Croft Road
Aldershot
Hants GU11 3HR
England

Ashgate Publishing Company
Old Post Road
Brookfield
Vermont 05036
USA

British Library Cataloguing in Publication Data

Robinson, David Keith
    Measuring forensic psychiatric and mental health nursing interactions
    1. Psychiatric nursing 2. Nurse and patient 3. Psychiatric nursing - Research 4. Nurse and patient - Research
    I. Title II. Reed, Val
    610. 7 ' 368

    ISBN 1 85972 221 0

Library of Congress Catalog Card Number: 96-84008

Printed and bound by Athenaeum Press, Ltd., Gateshead, Tyne & Wear.

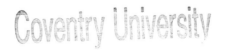

Contents

Figures and tables

Acknowledgements

The authors would like to acknowledge the following people:-

Patient and nurse participants within Rampton Hospital; Stanley Royd Hospital, Wakefield; Millbrook Mental Health Unit, Mansfield; and the Royal Liverpool Trust Hospital without whose kindness this study would not have been possible. Thanks are also extended to the many managers within all locations who assisted in negotiations regarding study venues and permissions for the study to proceed.

Margaret Owens; Ian Tennant; Christine Fisher; Michael Collins and Andrew Dean, who unstinctingly gave their considerable time and skills to collection of observational data. Peter Annets for technical assistance with the electronic database. Bridget Bower for providing administrative support.

Professors Justus Akinsanya and Val Reed for supervisory support. These dedicated people guided me through sometimes turbulent times with their special qualities to the completion of my PhD thesis on which this book is based.

My wife Averil Robinson, who stoically put up with considerable periods of domestic upheaval, especially during the analysis and writing up of the thesis and book!

Finally to John Thurgood and Senior Managers who have been instrumental in the application of findings to practice development.

David Robinson & Val Reed

Preface

Special Hospitals care for about 1500 patients and employ 3500 staff including doctors, nurses and teachers as well as other rehabilitation and ancillary staff. Patients not only suffer from varying mental health problems but are detained due to their dangerous and criminal propensities to either themselves or others. To date little has been documented about the complex nursing interactions between nursing staff and patients.

Several depth attempts at describing mainstream psychiatric care have been carried out but these are rapidly becoming outdated. This book offers a detailed account in a forensic psychiatric setting of nurse/patient interactions describing various elements of the care process. Because little was known about this population in relation to mainstream psychiatric services comparisons were made in order to understand the similarities and relationship. Some comparisons were also made with data of two decades ago and recent findings from general nursing contexts.

This therefore acts as a "first detailed account" of forensic care processes with implication for all other aspects of nursing care. Finally it breaks new ground in research methods contributing towards new health care and methodological knowledge.

1 Background and objectives

Purposes of care planning

The last two decades have seen increasing recognition of nurses' need to develop a problem-solving approach to their professional activities (Lamonica, 1979; Hunt, 1985). The resultant "nursing process" is concerned with making nursing care and treatment more systematic. The intention of care planning is to transform nursing into a research-based activity reliant upon empirical validation to a much greater extent than in the past (Aggleton and Chalmers, 1986).

Whilst numerous advantages have resulted from the introduction of individualised care (Kitson, 1986) this introduction has not been without its problems (Hayward, 1986, 1989; Robinson, 1990, 1990a). In discussing medical opinion Mitchell (1984) argues that, before nursing process activity can proceed, there needs to be an informed debate to distinguish between nursing process and the "processes of nursing".

Davis (1986b) points out that a significant feature of nurse education is to prepare nurses to approach individualised care. Quite clearly, if nurses do not receive appropriate education, then practice will not benefit as it should (Sheehan, 1991). In fact, almost a decade later, individualised care has still not been fully implemented. "A Vision for the Future" (Department of Health, 1993b) states clearly that "systems should be in place to encourage and facilitate development of individualised care. Where this is not the case, at least one pilot project should be in place and ready for evaluation by the end of the first year".

This statement implies that in many cases individualised care has still to be implemented. There need to be reliable and valid measures that can effectively describe the true impact of individualised care programmes (Denzin, 1970; Lorentzon, 1987).

The literature shows that there has been a steady output of papers concerning care implementation, measurement, and evaluation (e.g., Whitfield, 1989; Milne and Turton, 1986; Stephenson, 1984; Roper et al, 1983; Sheehan, 1989,1992; Robinson, 1990 & 1990a). Though some of the work has been empirically based, much of it has been based on largely untested, theoretical propositions rather than on empirically based studies. This leads to the assumption that there is still a dearth of observational evidence concerning practical impacts of the nursing process.

Nursing process as a key indicator of quality care

The pilot study (Robinson, 1988) helped to clarify fundamental links between nursing process and quality care, especially important since carers and consumers increasingly demand quality with individual care (cf e.g., Department of Health, 1989). The pilot study describes a number of findings which impact on the nature of future research. It shows that it is possible to describe the nature of nursing care observationally, in terms of nursing process and non-nursing process behaviours; and that the clinical characteristics of nursing care can be analysed in finer-grained qualitative detail than has been previously attempted, without loss of quantitative rigour. By using these methods it is possible to develop comparisons of documented and empirical care of considerable value in quality care studies. The instruments also possess generalising properties, making them potentially useful in wider multidisciplinary contexts of nursing care evaluation.

Qualitative indicators of quality care

Although the literature offers a steady output of papers examining theoretical content of each stage of the nursing process, these are seldom examined as empirical comparisons of care given with care planned (Hayward, 1986). Individualised care has frequently been described as a mere front or paper exercise. In Akinsanya's (1985) research examining the opinions of nurses turned doctors, one nurse comments: "... today the nurses are more likely to be sitting writing than actually nursing". This work supports an impression emergent from the pilot study (Robinson, 1988) that the largest proportion of nursing time is spent not interacting with patients.

The concept of nursing process as an indicator of quality has led to inclusion of the concept in a variety of measures. Lian (1985) describes nursing process as "the fundamental step towards quality assurance." During the last decade there has been a steady output of quality instruments to measure both nursing process and non-nursing process behaviours (cf, e.g., Hurst, 1988; Brooking, 1986, Goldstone, 1983, 1987). Whilst these take various forms including interviews, documentary audits and observational measures of care, few if any have adopted the detailed qualitative approach required to give precise details concerning observed processes of care. The application of fairly coarse-grained quantitative measures has reinforced a relatively static traditional design in quality studies, artificially limiting care analysis through lack of qualitative details which are necessary if outcomes are to be manipulated with any degree of precision.

Many definitions of quality exist. Mackie and Welch (1982) describe it as "a systematic approach for achieving the desired level of patient care." The importance of effective, adequately constructed research to assess the quality of care cannot be over-emphasised (Schmele, 1985). Without some form of adequate measurement or evaluation, nursing cannot aspire to any degree of precision; and individual patients will not benefit from continued improvements (Wilson-Barnett, 1986).

Concepts of quality

In the health service patients have a right to receive the best possible care (cf, e.g., DOH 1989abc, 1991, 1992, 1993ab). Since the launch of the strategy for nursing (DOH 1989b) nursing has had a potential impact in producing many innovations directly influencing the quality of patient care (Moores, 1993).

Quality is an issue of importance to all, whether in personal or professional life. The growth in personal and consumer awareness has placed considerable demands for defining and measuring concepts of quality (Shaw, 1986). Whilst notions and definitions of quality vary considerable depending on the context to be focused, attempts to discuss and define it are numerous within current literature (cf e.g., Ovretveit, 1990; Lorentzon, 1987; Hunt, 1990; Sines, 1989).

Ellis (1988) quotes the BSI definition of quality as "the totality of features or characteristics of a product service that bear on its ability to satisfy a given need"; and paraphrases it into more manageable form as "quality is that which gives complete customer satisfaction." Concern for quality has been considered fundamental to the practice of nursing, but only recently has the concept taken any systematic root (Green, et al 1991).

Whilst being part of industrial culture for some time quality assurance saw the first push in the United Kingdom in 1965, when the Royal College of Nursing established the first "Standards of Nursing Care" project. However it was not until the publication of two documents ("Standards of Nursing Care", RCN, 1980; "Towards Standards", RCN, 1981) that attempts were made to define with any degree of precision what actually constitutes high quality care. Since the underlying notion of quality assurance is systematically tomeasure aspects of service delivery (including nursing process), the last decade has seen an increase in methods designed to evaluate various aspects of service delivery. However Hunt (1990) notes a lack of consistency and coherence of the numerous quality studies reported in the literature that results in their rarely building upon one another. Shaw (1988) supports this, acknowledging there is "... little national consistency or coherence - let alone quality assurance in health care."

In considering quality of nursing care the researcher has to avoid the quest for a set of measures that will remain valid for all times (Lorentzon, 1987). In a changing world of health care policies such constant criteria are bound to fail. The quality assurance cycle of activity can be viewed as having three principal stages (Ellis, 1987).

The first stage is to observe practice and verify what is happening. The second stage is to compare this with what ought to be happening. The third stage is to implement appropriate change strategies.

Whilst concerned with the full cyclic approach, the present study begins by observing nursing practice to find out the precise details of the various care processes. Once the process of nursing is understood within the forensic psychiatric context, then suitable expectations of service delivery can be implemented through appropriate educational and resource management strategies.

Related issues in psychiatric settings

Thompson (1979) suggests that psychiatric nurses were taught in the past to do rather than think; and to accept rather than question. Recent evidence shows that nurses do not follow a systematic, problem-solving approach to patient care (cf, e.g., Hurst and Dean, 1987; Tanner, 1987). Whether this is due to inimical nurse education or to some fault in the "process" model of clinical problem-solving has yet to be resolved. In organisational terms, the almost breathless rate of change occurring in nursing has led to a lack of the gradualistic attributes of major change (Robinson, 1988). As a result the nursing process was seized upon and promulgated intensively and power-coercively, with scant regard to fundamental underlying issues such as educational preparation (Sheehan, 1989); social climate of change; staff perceptions of the process; the need to implement such changes in a carefully phased normative-reeducative management context (Ashworth, 1985); the need for repeated evaluation and systematic enquiry into its implementation (Robertson, 1981); and for continuing support to improve both knowledge and skills in delivering individual patient care (Aggleton and Chalmers, 1986).

If effective change strategies continue to be ignored then quality issues will suffer in a similar manner and will be little further on after a decade of implementation. There is then likely to be "too much investment to let go" (Hardy and Engel, 1987).

In specialties where psychological needs and problems often assume a greater priority for intervention than physical needs, the psychiatric nursing disciplines have important specific problems in implementing individualised care programmes (Barrowclough et al, 1984; Whyte and Youhill, 1984). The implications for forensic psychiatric nursing, where patients are dangerous both to themselves and others, cause still more concern.

The challenge of nursing in psychiatric settings is formidable, in that it is easy for staff to become unwittingly over-protective and custodial: and nurses may well find themselves inadvertently slipping back into the task-oriented routines of the institutional days (Willard, 1984). This is especially so in the case of dangerous patients, since added security in the prevention of patients' harming themselves or others may set difficulties in providing the right balance of therapy against security.

Findings from related studies

As nursing strives for quality care, consumers and health authorities are demanding the assurance of quality care linked with individualised care planning (Gould, 1985). Periodically, disquieting findings emerge. Thus in a recent quality audit undertaken into psychiatric nursing care, there is evidence to suggest that individualised care in some contexts may still be largely a paper exercise: and that nurses do not follow the systematic model of planned delivery of individual care posited by nursing theorists (Hurst and Dean, 1987; Tanner, 1987). This is perhaps scarcely surprising, given considerable educational deficits including lack of tutorial support for students (Davis, 1983).

There is also evidence to suggest that in some psychiatric contexts nurses spend approximately two-and-a-half times as long in the ward office as in direct care of patients (Cormack, 1976; Street, 1982; Hurst, 1987, 1992). Street (1982) goes further by stating that some nurses were seen not to interact with patients for considerable periods; whilst Cormack (1976) notes that the clinical expertise of the ward charge nurse was wasted because of the burden of administrative and clerical duties.

Furthermore, whilst the charge nurse rarely interacted with patients, s/he was seen as valuable to them. A further relevant issue was that nurses on average spent only approximately thirteen per cent of their time talking to patients. In a more recent study (Cormack, 1983) there was identification of a "lack of time to talk" to patients by nursing staff; a lack of ward teaching; and the amount of nursing time spent on domestic duties also gave cause for concern.

Finally, in a recent quality audit of care, Hurst and Howard (1988) show that direct care to patients accounted for approximately 25 per cent of activity; with individualised care accounting for considerably less. These findings were supported within the pilot context of the present study (Robinson, 1988). If such observations are supported within the present study, then these findings may impact directly on the quality of patient care. The present study describes a detailed search for effective methods of carrying out care evaluation linked to nursing process within a forensic environment. If long-standing care deficits, first observed more than a decade ago, are confirmed by this study, there may well be substantial implications for introducing change into the static scenario of psychiatric nursing care.

Recent data from extensive studies carried out within general nursing showed that nurses spent between thirty-five and forty-five percent of their time giving indirect patient care, thus taking considerable time and nursing skills away from the bedside (Department of Health, 1988; Hurst, 1992). Rhys-Hearn (1979a) supports this finding by noting that activities observed within one ward compared well with those observed in other units, despite differences in structure and resourcing. Similar studies show that levels of direct care are falling (cf, e.g., Hilton, 1985; Hurst, 1992; Hurst and Quinn, 1992). If found within the present study, such low levels of direct nursing care have interesting implications for the future of forensic psychiatric nursing care, given the findings of the pilot study (Robinson, 1988).

Patient involvement

The failure of nurses in psychiatric settings positively to define their role may have contributed considerably to difficulties in rehabilitating patients and in overcoming identified problems (Mackie and Welch, 1982). Without a clear perception of her role the nurse may well find that the patient is still being fitted into traditional institutional care regimes with the attendant depersonalisation so often evident (Kitson, 1986; Thompson, 1979). The philosophical basis for nursing is concerned with enabling the individual to achieve and maintain optimum physical, psychological and social well-being

(Department of Health, 1993b); yet the patient is still frequently excluded from involvement in his/her own care. Where s/he is included, nurses have often cared for the "average" patient rather than for the markedly unique individual (Davies, 1981).

In the field of mental health the evaluation of quality has been a particularly difficult area because of the frequently expressed attitude that "... it's no good asking the consumers (patients) their points of view because they are too ill" (Green, 1987). Today, there is a shift in view. Whether ill or not, those in hospital have views about the quality of service they receive and the quality of life they endure (Hunt, 1987). Recent dramatic changes in the health care professions and in consumer participation have increased the concern to promote quality assurance and involve the patient in working towards meeting those needs (Sines, 1989a). In particular the involvement of patients in satisfaction studies and surveys has become relatively common (Whitfield and Baker, 1992). "We need to take into account what a person wishes or desires" (Donabedian, 1993). Unfortunately some professionals take the view that patient involvement in consumer audit, as well as auditing in general, are still an "add-on" to practice and not a regular part of the everyday care of patients (Pringle, 1992).

To achieve more individualised inputs and improved nurse/patient partnerships, clinical leaders, together with managers, may have to reconsider the way work is organised and how care is given to patients (Department of Health, 1993b). Little can be done without research that informs us of exactly what happens in specific nursing contexts; systematically describing nursing practice so that resource management decisions and improved care practices can be carried out.

Auditing in quality

It is expected that this study will contribute empirical evidence towards the development of valid and reliable indicators of quality that can be used for quality audit. As yet few investigations into the relationship between quality and individualised care have been undertaken within the context of the Special Hospitals. Psychiatric settings present added problems in evaluating planned individual care; and require more empirical studies to investigate its implementation (Bowman, 1983; Ashworth, 1985).

There has been much pressure to undertake audit, especially from political sources (Baker, 1993). For good practice to be commissioned, it is essential that it is properly analysed, documented and disseminated. Target Three (Department of Health, 1993b) relates to the general consensus in the health care professions that providing patient care on an individual basis, and developing and establishing monitoring and audit systems in order to determine the "foundation stones" of a high quality service, are essential. Another important aspect of this report relates to further health care promotion: "... in order to deliver high quality care, nurses should ensure that their work is research-based, represents good practice, and is accurately and clearly documented."

Never before has there been such a need for, or interest in, measuring what nurses and other health care professionals do (Dickson, 1987). "Audits can work to improve (practitioner) behaviour and bring it more in line with professional standards, to the extent that they have been validated by science." (Donabedian, 1993).

Summary of pilot study

The pilot study built on earlier, pioneering work in observational methodology (King, Raynes and Tizard, 1971; Reed, 1978); and on theoretical links existing between nursing process and clinical quality care (cf., e.g., Lian, 1985; Brooking, 1986; Hurst, 1987; Hurst and Dean, 1987). Using specially-designed interview, observation and documentary analytic schedules, it described nursing care within an assessment unit at Rampton Hospital; and analysed staff and patient perceptions of nursing care (Robinson, 1988). It sought to characterise one psychiatric nursing care setting, whilst obtaining data about attitudes to nursing process from patients, nurses and other care staff. Research instruments were designed to possess generalising properties for use in subsequent, related quality care studies.

During the pilot, seventeen nurses and eleven patients on an assessment unit were observed during a five-week period. Observations of eleven nursing care plans, and interviews with patients, nurses and non-nursing staff were carried out. Externally-based pilot observations and documentary analyses were followed by main ward observations using random rotational time-sampling techniques. Documentation of care planning and recording were rated on an analytic checklist. Face and content validity of instruments were supported by clinical and academic informants. Inter-rater reliability was field-tested using synchronous observations on selected data sets; with mean documentary and observational reliability coefficients of 0.83 and 0.87 respectively.

Analysis of pilot study data showed that patient care was largely supervisory, with little individual care. Comparisons with analogous data from external contexts showed similar patterns. Approximately 50 per cent of observations were of administrative duties. Relief nurses were unable to give continuity of care equivalent to that given by regular members of the ward team. Observational data were analysed for staff interactions with patients. Up to 73 per cent of observed behaviours were of indirect patient care; with only 18-26 per cent spent in direct contact with patients. Care plan documentation showed a relatively well-developed version of care planning was in use: but there were anomalous areas, including in some cases lack of patient assessment; no prioritisation of needs; and late evaluation.

Findings from pilot study

The pilot study describes a number of potentially important findings which impact on the nature of future research. Among other findings it shows: that it is possible to describe the nature of nursing care observationally in terms of nursing process and non-nursing process behaviours; that the clinical characteristics of such nursing care can be analysed in more precise qualitative detail than has previously been attempted, without loss of quantitative rigour; that, using the above methods, it is possible to develop comparisons of documented and empirical care of considerable potential benefit in developmental qualitative studies; and that the instruments used possess generalising properties making them potentially useful in wider, multidisciplinary contexts of nursing care evaluation.

The pilot findings further indicated that positive staff attitudes to nursing process were likely to provide support for related quality assurance evaluation programmes. Educative strategies in care planning, communication and therapies clearly needed development; and a preliminary package of change was sketched out (cf Robinson, 1988, pp 204-223).

Review of current quality methods

Whilst there is a growing number of quality measures emerging, there are several methods that are now in substantial use. Similarly, whilst these methods are used in many adaptations at local level, it is important to review them because of their influential nature and the need to overcome potential methodological limitations. Whilst this section reviews selected, recently implemented quality methods relating directly to this study, it does not take into account such approaches to quality as medical audit (Shaw, 1989) or DySSSy ("dynamic standard setting system", Kitson, 1990); though the researcher recognises these as useful and legitimate frameworks for the improvement of professional quality.

The Rush-Medicus project

The Medicus Systems Corporation of Chicago, in collaboration with its clients and with the influence of certain nurse scheduling systems (Hegyvary and Haussmann, 1976) carried out extensive research examining a large number of instruments concerned with measuring the quality of care. Amongst several problems identified with these methods was that of the definition of nursing duties. Following extensive piloting in twenty-one hospitals, the resulting Rush-Medicus System took the form of a master list of 220 items to be scored as a standard expected of an experienced registered nurse.

These are structured within the four elements of the nursing process. The larger proportion of items refers to patient care; the rest to various features of the unit. Data are collected by sampled observations, interview and documentary audits. Although intended for wide application, its scope was actually limited to medical, surgical and paediatric areas (Balogh, 1991).

Monitor

Monitor is an adaptation from the Rush-Medicus nursing process methodology (Goldstone, 1987). Monitor seeks to make explicit criteria which are implicit in the quality statements of nurses and relies on aspects of nursing that are observable as having occurred or not. It is based on research which demonstrated that there are aspects of care which can be observed (Hegyvary and Haussmann, 1976).

Monitor is based on the nursing process and consists of two hundred criterion items. Each criterion demands observations to which the response is usually yes or no. A trained nurse observer using fifteen-minute time-sampling techniques obtains information on the ward to establish a picture of policies, staffing levels, procedures and support services. Patients are classified according to dependency and nursing observations are carried out to record activities. Observations are made against predetermined criteria; hence the mainly quantitative nature of the instrument. Goldstone (1987) writes: "... the only abilities required to score Monitor are the abilities to count and calculate percentages." (p 68).

Central Notts psychiatric nursing audit (CNPNA)

The structure of CNPNA was devised by Hurst and Howard, 1988, using the principles of criteria for care (Ball and Goldstone, 1983) and Monitor (Goldstone, Ball and Collier, 1983), which were themselves adapted from the Rush-Medicus system and utilised a nursing process approach. The structure

10

of the audit is threefold, consisting of a patient dependency rating scale; a nursing activity analysis based upon external observations; and a "quality patient care scale" based upon the nursing process.

Although similar to the previously mentioned instruments, CNPNA is specifically designed to incorporate psychiatric activities. Again, observational data types are determined largely by the quantitative design of the audit; and nursing activities are recorded against predetermined criteria using ten-minute time-sampling techniques. Observational data are collected by time-sampling techniques and determine the amount and type of work done by nurses. The "quality patient care scale" examines the completeness of care given to patients through the nursing process framework as reflected in the documentation.

Quality of patient care scale (Qualpacs)

The Quality of Patient Care Scale was designed to measure the standard of nursing care that is received by the patient or patients. Designed in America, Qualpacs was constructed using the Slater performance rating scale (1967) as its theoretical base (Wandelt and Stewart, 1975). The Slater scale evaluates the competence of the individual nurse as she is observed in the various care processes with patients. Performance is measured against a given standard which is provided by the scale. This is then measured using a seven-point, Likert-type scale consisting of "poorest" care through to "best" care. Data collection and analysis are mainly quantitative in nature. Observational data are collected against predetermined categories using randomly selected patients over a two-hour period.

The eighty-four items within the Slater Scale that were used to judge the performance of the nurse were reworded to apply to the patient. Additional items were added and unsuitable ones disused. Qualpacs (Wandelt and Ager, 1978) assesses the quality of care provided by the ward or unit; but not that given by individual nurses. Assessors evaluate the nursing received by a sample of patients and that standard is regarded as a reflection of nursing care to all patients on the ward. The process of nursing is scrutinised through direct observation and assessment of nursing records. Scores are allocated to every observable action.

Phaneuf nursing audit

Phaneuf's nursing audit is a survey method for evaluating nursing care through detailed observational examination of the patient's nursing records (Lesnik and Anderson, 1955). Phaneuf constructed fifty descriptive statements of nursing actions related to the patient. These checklist items are applied against the nursing documentation and scored on a three-point scale (yes, no, uncertain).

Phaneuf's (1976) assumption is that the records will faithfully represent the care that is given (Bradshaw, 1987); and that the higher the scores obtained, the better the care received by patients.

Nursing process measurement scale

The nursing process Measurement Scale was developed as part of a PhDstudy investigating patient and family participation in nursing care (Brooking, 1986). Although two main instruments were designed within the study, these were used to develop a nurse's self-rating scale to measure key activities of the nursing process. Several hundred books and articles were examined to identify statements which described practical use of the nursing process (Brooking, 1988). Most of the available literature was American and as a result required the adaptation and validation of independent British nurses. As a result of this, sixty-five items emerged which were classified into categories of assessment; nursing diagnosis; planning; implementation; and evaluation.

Following external validation and testing, a final forty-three items were found to be valid indicators of the practical use of the nursing process. Preliminary work in the methodological development used the items as interview and observation schedules to assess nursing process components carried out in eight wards, half of which were not using the nursing process. Although observations of nursing process were completed, these were centred on determining if eleven of the pre-selected criteria were present, rather than measuring to what extent nursing process activities were happening compared with other activities.

The resultant instrument was a ward nurse's self-rating scale that required nurses to respond to the thirty-seven items on a six-point scale, according to what extent the item was being carried out. The method has a variety of uses and can be used as an audit tool by clinical nurses to examine their own practices, and as a quality assessment in nursing within the structure-process-outcome model of evaluation.

The scale has not yet been subject to criticism as far as can be established; and appears to have been successfully applied to several clinical settings (Smith, 1986a; Harris, 1987). There is no doubt that the theoretical testing within the development stages through the process of research has influenced considerably the reliabilities and validities that have been obtained.

Potential benefits of the present study

Potential benefits from a descriptive study of indicators of quality care are considerable. It will contribute to current understanding and evaluation; and to the encouragement and promotion of further evaluative work. The present study will provide a clear conceptualisation of care processes as carried out within a Special Hospital, as well as within selected external settings within the NHS; giving insights into current strengths and weaknesses. As a practical spin-off, it is expected that the study will provide numerous insights calculated to improve present levels of quality care. It will further provide scientific data for the development of quality audits and extended follow-up studies, as well as developmental features for initiating other research.

The study will permit an analysis of social change by which implementation was introduced and developed at Rampton Hospital. The impact of these strategies can be examined by means of various indices (e.g., staff knowledge and perceptions of, and attitudes towards, individual processes of care): and inferences drawn regarding future potentially successful clinical, educational and management strategies. It is anticipated that this research will contribute towards new descriptive methods of enquiry; describe some central elements of the nature of forensic psychiatric care; and contribute new knowledge relating to its various care processes.

Finally, few investigators have yet demonstrated to their peers the effects of individualised care in terms of patient outcomes within forensic psychiatric care, though this type of study is the ideal (Hayward, 1986). Whilst a patient outcomes study is beyond the scope of this inquiry, it is hoped that it will yield data regarding potentially useful indices and further possible development in that area.

Research objectives

The present study therefore builds on traditional quantitative methods of data recording and analysis; but additionally uses a detailed qualitative/descriptive approach without loss of quantitative rigour. Whilst adopting some of the principles of Donabedian (1966), in his analysis of structures, processes and outcomes of care, the methods specifically examine processes of care in a way that has not so far been undertaken by other methods. The objectives of the study are to: (1) revise and validate research instruments used in the pilot for general use in quality care studies; (2) utilise these to obtain baseline values of nursing care for use in systematic evaluation; (3) examine the status of nursing care and documentation in the selected care settings; (4) describe nurse/patient perceptions of, and attitudes towards, individual care; (5) compare and contrast data obtained from internal and external psychiatric care settings; (6) and assess implications of these data for further research.

2 Theoretical approaches

Anthropological and philosophical issues

This study is approached from several linked perspectives which form the basis for a close and detailed study of human beings. Qualitative research methods provide an important component in enabling clinicians to discover, describe, document and understand the subtle attributes that make people the unique beings that they are (Carter, 1985). The growing importance of understanding empirical phenomena of specific interest to nursing has become the rationale for developing nursing on a scientific basis (Leininger, 1979; Newman, 1979; Rogers, 1979; Watson, 1979).

Firstly, the anthropological quest has been to understand the ways of human beings through creative qualitative methodology which has led to "meaningful and refreshing new discoveries about human beings in the world today" (Leininger, 1992). Anthropology is a descriptive science because of its basic method of describing characteristics of human behaviours (Osborne, 1973; Davis, 1984; Carter, 1985). Therefore, anthropological methods are particularly useful when describing what nurses do and the reactions that patients have to interactions. However, the researcher has to avoid the problem of possibly eliciting more information than is required or intended (Davis, 1986a).

Descriptive observations can therefore assist in collecting first-hand information about nursing activity (Akinsanya, 1986a). This approach is useful since, as far as the writers are aware, no one has yet attempted systematically to describe nursing care as given within the relevant forensic psychiatric services. Unless otherwise stated, the present study relates to this specialised service context; although wider psychiatric care practices are discussed and reviewed. Approaches using descriptive observation techniques allow the researcher to "live and capture" life experiences of the nurses and patients under

14

study (McCaugherty, 1992a). Subsequent translation of these findings into care constructs (categories) will allow meaningful interpretation of data and cross-cultural comparisons (Kleinman, 1987).

Secondly, a phenomenological approach allows the "description" of the phenomena under study as experienced both by patients and nursing staff (Carter, 1985). The goal of empirical phenomenological research is systematically to examine life situations and human experience: for example, the situations which patients find themselves in (Lynch-Sauer, 1985). In addition it describes the world as experienced by the participants in order that qualitative analysis can uncover common meanings (Baker et al, 1992). This approach strives to ensure that the researcher is free from preconceived notions, allowing theories to emerge and be generated within the empirical context, rather than relying solely on predetermined theory and related testing (Glaser and Strauss, 1967).

The phenomenological approach can be particularly useful by "transforming" a person's experiences into actions and language (Reinhartz, 1983). It enables the researcher to conceptualise the person's original experience; allows the transformation of understanding of the original experience into conceptual categories; and permits the researcher to transform these categories into some form of written document which can then be used to clarify and highlight new experiences (Leininger, 1975).

Qualitative methods are valuable to help generate new theories; but more importantly their clear advantage over quantitative methods is that of generating "thick (detailed) descriptions of, and rich insights concerning, unknown or vaguely-known phenomena" (Leininger, 1992). In this case we refer to the "vaguely-known" characteristics of forensic psychiatric nursing care. The goals of qualitative research are not necessarily to measure something and generalise (Lincoln et al, 1985); but rather to understand the phenomena under study and offer rich accounts of what happens/is happening, thus unveiling the nature, essence and characteristics of the phenomena as fully as possible.

Qualitative studies also possess an important feature whereby one can use the findings to improve human conditions whilst still conducting the study, as well as testing out early developing theories (Leininger, 1987; Reason, 1989).

In action research based and qualitative studies, there is a developmental issue where it is not always necessary to wait for the study to be completed before findings can be used. Regular discussions with participants throughout the study, as well as regular dissemination, ensure developmental features.

Finally, the use of multi-methods in a study more accurately to depict the phenomena under investigation (e.g., observational techniques; documentary analysis; and questioning) can, at its best, materially assist in cross-validation of findings.

15

Relationship between theory and practice

Using these approaches to carry out nursing research helps understanding of the phenomena under study. However, the application of theory in practice can often be a cause for concern (Alexander, 1983; McCaugherty, 1990). Which comes first: research or theory? The present study uses existing theoretical frameworks (cf Leininger's conceptual theory-generating model, 1986). Riehl and Roy (1980) describe theory as "as scientific, acceptable general principle, which governs practice or is proposed to explain observed facts", and is furthermore used to "describe, explain and predict part of the empirical world".

The nature of the relationship between theory and practice is dependent on two variables; education and practice (Rafferty, 1992). Education is affected by factors such as the educational setting; quality and methods of teaching and curriculum; and its interpretation. Practice issues relate to the environment in which nursing care is given; and to the skills, knowledge and attitudes of practitioners.

Reliance on the spoken and written word alone seem to present a barrier for nurses implementing research findings into practice (McCaugherty, 1992b). A recurring question concerning nursing research in recent years has been directed to the usefulness and relevance of its theories and findings in practice (Akinsanya, 1988; Stanton and Crotty, 1991). This is further supported by Sheehan (1986) who states that applying theory generated from research is one of the biggest challenges that nurses face today. Smith (1986) urges the profession to implement nursing research findings; and maintains that most research has at least one finding that can be applied to practice. However, much further debate is required if nurses are systematically to generate and utilise theory (Draper 1992).

Using anthropological and phenomenological approaches helps the researcher "live and capture" the life experiences of patients and carers, as well as observe behaviour which will facilitate and help develop integration of theories into care practice (McCaugherty, 1992).

Akinsanya (1984) points out the substantial evidence suggesting that theory has a clarifying effect on practice: yet nurses still remain distant from, and suspicious of, theories of nursing. Involving nurses in carrying out research, as well as simply participating in it, can serve to improve understanding and help bridge the "theory-practice gap". Use of detailed descriptive accounts of the various processes of nursing can enhance nurses' attitudes towards improving care as well as understanding their unique roles. More research (the critical factor in knowing and explaining) is required if we are to understand care in-depth (Leininger, 1990).

Concepts of caring: research contribution

Concepts of caring have been among the least-studied areas of human knowledge. Until the last decade the nursing profession has rarely studied care systematically in relation to nursing (Leininger, 1978, 1992). Knowledge needs to be developed from both the emic (insider's) and the etic (outsider's) perspectives, underpinned by empirical work focusing on descriptive and philosophical methods (McFarland, 1990). In addition empirical evidence needs to embrace a variety of paradigmatic approaches that advance methodologies through creative thinking.

There are aspects of caring behaviour which uniquely distinguish nursing from the contributions of other disciplines (Leininger, 1984). It is necessary empirically to explain and understand the roles of caregiver and care recipient if nurses are to preserve and maintain these aspects of effective care (Leininger, 1981). Only when these roles are systematically examined will understanding and definition occur to any degree.

Questions have been posed in relation to what nurses should be doing, and what constitutes a successful nurse (Nicholas, 1969). Unless nurses can understand their roles and the processes of care they deliver, there will remain a lack of planned nursing care and nursing objectives resulting in an inability to evaluate the quality of care (Lambersten, 1965). "Where nursing cultures do not have individualism, there will be limited signs of self-practice and more signs of other care practices such as task-orientated care." (Leininger, 1985).

Requirement to generate and test nursing theory

Nursing theory currently emphasises the importance of, and need for, further research; and the centrality of the continuing process of refining theoretical beliefs. A popular contemporary theory relates to the need of the nurse researcher to obtain qualitative, documented, descriptive accounts of observed and verified behaviour that reveal the essence, nature, process and attributes of caring behaviour and therapeutic nursing care within a culture (Leininger, 1978). This approach requires careful consideration in relation to all nursing studies if the profession is to continue to develop substantive nursing knowledge.

There are four broad reasons for studying care (Leininger, 1981):

1   the construct of care is critical to human growth, development and survival;
2   it is necessary to explain and understand the roles of caregiver and care recipient;

3   to preserve and maintain care is essential for survival through time;
4   the nursing profession has rarely systematically studied care in relation to nursing care.

Leininger's work has led to the generation of numerous theories, some of which concern the present study. In particular she posits a theory-generating model which is discussed later. Her propositions support the need for further research and for the continuing process of refining theoretical beliefs.

Leininger (1984) refers to qualitative research as "methods and techniques for observing, documenting, analyzing and interpreting attributes, patterns, characteristics, and meanings of specific features under study." Here the main feature is documentation and description of the phenomena. Quantitative research focuses on objective analysis of discrete and pre-selected variables that can be measured against each other. In addition there is a strong manipulation of data rarely if ever present in qualitative types of research. The various care processes cannot be measured so precisely in instrumental terms. Careful documentation and description are required to reflect the true nature of the care aspect. However, data collection itself does not answer research questions. The research data need to be analyzed in an organised systematic way, by means of which trends and relationships can be developed from the data (Polit and Hungler, 1989).

A conceptual theory-generating model

A conceptual theory-generating model, which involves three phases in obtaining and analyzing data to generate nursing theory, has been used here as the paradigm to develop study methods and related hypotheses (Leininger, 1986: see Figure 1, and "transformational" model, Figure 2):

PHASE 1: The systematic study and classification of nursing care beliefs, values and practices, as cognitively perceived within a designated culture *(ethnonursing)*. This identifies the major sources used to derive *emic* (local) and *etic* (external) issues related to psychiatric nursing care. Firstly, nurse interactions and behaviours are observed and studied. Secondly, the social-structural features, such as educational, management and clinical implications, are examined. Thirdly, the cultural attitudes and perceptions of nursing staff and patients regarding care are investigated. Finally, health care systems such as care planning documentation are reviewed, and their relationship to empirical components of care established.

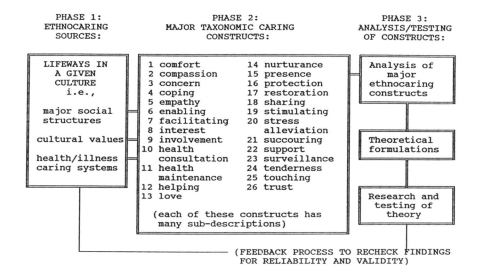

PHASE 1: ETHNOCARING SOURCES:	PHASE 2: MAJOR TAXONOMIC CARING CONSTRUCTS:	PHASE 3: ANALYSIS/TESTING OF CONSTRUCTS:

LIFEWAYS IN A GIVEN CULTURE i.e.,

major social structures

cultural values

health/illness caring systems

1 comfort	14 nurturance
2 compassion	15 presence
3 concern	16 protection
4 coping	17 restoration
5 empathy	18 sharing
6 enabling	19 stimulating
7 facilitating	20 stress
8 interest	alleviation
9 involvement	21 succouring
10 health	22 support
consultation	23 surveillance
11 health	24 tenderness
maintenance	25 touching
12 helping	26 trust
13 love	

(each of these constructs has many sub-descriptions)

Analysis of major ethnocaring constructs

Theoretical formulations

Research and testing of theory

(FEEDBACK PROCESS TO RECHECK FINDINGS FOR RELIABILITY AND VALIDITY)

Figure 1   Leininger's conceptual theory generating model (after Leininger, 1986)

PHASE 2: involves classifying observational data into care constructs or behaviours.   Observations of care are carefully examined and similar interactions/behaviours categorised to enable measurement. This enables the development of care constructs that relate directly to the emic culture as well as indicating similarities in terms of the etic factors.

PHASE 3: involves the analysis and testing of the care constructs previously identified which relate to both emic and etic issues. From these data research hypotheses are developed and tested and subsequent nursing theory generated. The model then returns to Phase One and continues its cyclic approach.

Thus the "transformational" model appears as follows:

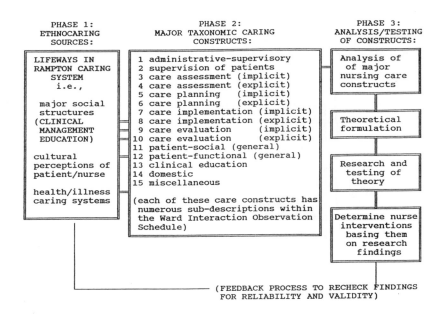

PHASE 1: ETHNOCARING SOURCES:	PHASE 2: MAJOR TAXONOMIC CARING CONSTRUCTS:	PHASE 3: ANALYSIS/TESTING OF CONSTRUCTS:
LIFEWAYS IN RAMPTON CARING SYSTEM i.e., major social structures (CLINICAL MANAGEMENT EDUCATION) cultural perceptions of patient/nurse health/illness caring systems	1 administrative-supervisory 2 supervision of patients 3 care assessment (implicit) 4 care assessment (explicit) 5 care planning (implicit) 6 care planning (explicit) 7 care implementation (implicit) 8 care implementation (explicit) 9 care evaluation (implicit) 10 care evaluation (explicit) 11 patient-social (general) 12 patient-functional (general) 13 clinical education 14 domestic 15 miscellaneous (each of these care constructs has numerous sub-descriptions within the Ward Interaction Observation Schedule)	Analysis of of major nursing care constructs Theoretical formulation Research and testing of theory Determine nurse interventions basing them on research findings

(FEEDBACK PROCESS TO RECHECK FINDINGS
FOR RELIABILITY AND VALIDITY)

Figure 2   Relationship of Leininger's theoretical model to present study

Quality health care studies

Quality health care studies to date have been diverse. Different methods emerging over the last three decades indicate the difficulty experienced in measuring the concept of quality. According to Schmadl (1979) the purpose of quality assurance is to ensure the patient a specified degree of excellence through continuous measurement and evaluation.

Until recently health care systems have been relatively closed because they have tended to be largely controlled and regulated by specific groups such as the medical profession (Leininger, 1975). Although a start has been made, nursing still needs to bring about a substantial research effort to enable the impact of nursing changes in the health care system (cf, e.g., Bryant, 1975). Such initiatives need to be built upon solid groundwork of careful observation carried out within sound theoretical frameworks.

As a consequence of nursing's past reliance on quantitative research models (Field and Morse, 1985), designs have tended to be relatively reductionist and static. This has artificially limited the growth of nursing knowledge, tending to lead to naive applications of the scientific model to nursing research (Leininger, 1975). The Rush-Medicus System (Hegyvary, 1976) has been a classic example, originally developed for management purposes with traditional frequency recording in data collection.

Donabedian's threefold classification of structure, process, outcome is implicit within all methodologies; but most measures concentrate on structure and process (Donabedian, 1966). Whilst outcome studies are becoming more common, few if any tackle the real problem of forensic care outcomes: that is, whether patients actually get better as a result of specific care inputs within forensic psychiatric nursing (Simpson, 1989; Hughes, 1991; Burrow, 1992).

The two main methods currently used in qualitative data collection are, firstly, the auditing of nurses' notes based on the assumption that good and complete nursing notes reflect quality of care (Phaneuf, 1976; Brooking, 1988); and secondly, the obtaining of observational measures to determine whether or not a nurse has performed specific tasks in connection with patient care (Wandelt and Stewart; 1975 Hegyvary and Haussmann, 1976). However, recent authors suggest that chart audit is open to criticism, in that much care may be given that is not recorded. Similarly, care may be recorded but not actually given (cf, e.g., Barnett and Wainwright, 1987).

Dissatisfaction with current quality measures

Despite considerable testing-out of quality methods, often with substantive research input, the last few years have seen an increasing number of articles critically reviewing current systems.

The current literature reveals issues such as: doubts about validity and reliability (Smith, 1986); lack of inter-rater reliability and difficulty in splitting interactions into sub-components of care (Barnett and Wainwright, 1987); forcing of complex nursing activities into inappropriate quantitative measures (Dickson, 1987); quantitative forcing of nursing interactions and lack of validity; (Redfern and Norman, 1990); ten-minute time-sampling and researcher interference (Balogh, 1991); complexity of defining levels of activity and poor inter-rater reliability (Oliver, 1991); measurement techniques requiring much development (West, 1991); and artificial forcing of interactions and disruption of ward staff (Tomalin, 1991). However, it should be borne in mind that these weaknesses are noted with equal frequency in attempted adaptations as in the original models.

Current weaknesses

Validity of care constructs or criteria seems to be one of the main critical issues, especially in adapted methods (Brittle and Marsh, 1986; Barnett and Wainwright, 1987; Whelan, 1987; Hilton and Dawson, 1988; Redfern and

Norman, 1990). Validity of criteria is often established on the grounds that they are aligned to a particular model of nursing such as the nursing process or the methods from which it is adapted. Openshaw (1984) notes that, in fact, it is unknown whether or not the nursing process does result in improved patient care. It is this premise which undergirds a whole range of untested assumptions underlying the notion of measuring care. It is quite clear that nurses are implementing methods for quality measurement assuming that they are built on sound theoretical testing, and their practical application to the setting. Even if such premises are true, then once adaptations are made, extensive retesting for validity is required.

Barnett and Wainwright (1981) point out that the Phaneuf nursing record audit has little use within the United Kingdom; and where it has, it lacks both validity and reliability. Other authors such as Bradshaw (1987) reflect on its use more creatively. Similarly, MONITOR reportedly lacks validity; and it is questioned whether or not there is appropriate evidence of inter-rater reliabilities. Smith (1986) casts considerable doubt on whether use of QUALPACS in the United Kingdom is reliable and valid. Ventura et al (1989) point out that, because of the complexity of nursing, it is difficult to define and measure appropriately. Redfern and Norman (1990) go further by stating that ".... most instruments are in need of extensive validity testing in relationship to what they purport to measure.": a state of affairs which must cast doubt on the soundness of their theoretical bases.

Reliance on American methods appears to cause considerable concern to the developers of British measures. Whilst it has been established that there are similar nursing values, beliefs and approaches to care in the United States (Marriner, 1986), cultural differences exist which must reflect in the nature and type of care delivery and consequently in its measurement. Brooking (1986) notes that a review of American literature failed to reveal objective indicators or criteria against which the use of the nursing process could be quantified, despite systems already being in use and supposedly measuring aspects of it (cf, eg, Phaneuf; Rush-Medicus; QUALPACS).

Regarding observational methods, there appears to be one main theme emerging from the current literature surrounding quality measurement. Recent studies indicate that there is little evidence of clear assumptions on which these are based (Balogh, 1991). Problems encountered with such methods have been related to ten-minute time-sampling of nurse activity. This has resulted in different care activities being emphasised. Consequently, such methods fail to provide a true reflection of the range of complicated interactions in which nurses are involved. Similarly in Psychiatric Audit, the disruption of nursing activities caused by observers seeking to clarify what they were doing appears to have a negative effect on nursing staff.

Although observations are measured against pre-set criteria, many interactions have implications for several categories, resulting in possible confusion and artificial forcing of observations into criterial categories. Tomalin (1991) supports this view, stating that MONITOR suffers from this problem as well as from ambiguities in the interpretation of questions and answers. Similarly, Oliver (1991) and Wainwright (1987) suggest that identifying interactions within QUALPACS, and having to break these down into sub-components and then rate them is a complex problem, in addition to that of achieving acceptable levels of rating between observers.

It is scarcely surprising that current quality measures suffer from these problems, since most observational measures originated from, or were influenced by, similar sources. Similarly, the forcing of complex nursing activities into pre-determined care constructs through quantitative recording has limited use. Redfern and Norman (1990) report a reliance on measures that attempt to translate complex nurse-patient interactions into items and scores. Dickson (1987) supports this by casting doubt on whether any system can arrive at finely-tuned figures. West (1991) concludes that much work is required further to develop audit techniques.

There seems to be a design stasis which has resulted in determining pre-set standards of care or criteria against which observations are measured. Results from these data types can only be determined in frequency or percentage form. In other words, there is no way that they can be interrogated qualitatively. It is clear that there has been a traditional fault in seeking to adapt quantitative measurement to analyses which should logically be more qualitative in nature.

New, or refined, quality instruments are needed which accurately evaluate the quality of care given and provide pertinent data that can be used to improve nursing practice (Curtis, 1985). In addition the unfortunate lack of coherence of quality studies - which rarely build upon one another - further indicates the continuing need to improve methods (Shaw, 1988).

Current observational methods

Figure 3 identifies the quality measures that have influenced the current study.

Two main observational measures are used: that of *direct observational audit*, examining staff/staff and staff/patient interactions; and that of *documentary audit*, examining the completeness of related nursing documentation.

The figure shows the methods which influenced the two observational measures used in the present study. Building on these methods, the current study seeks to show that it is possible to integrate both quantitative and qualitative assessments to analyze psychiatric nursing care. The study offers an essentially qualitative approach, but without prejudice to the importance of quantitative methods, which are also used. Little is known about the precise details of the various care processes in psychiatric and forensic psychiatric care; and qualitative methods are particularly useful when describing phenomena from the emic perspective; that is, from the point of view of the actors concerned (Field and Morse, 1985; Leininger, 1975).

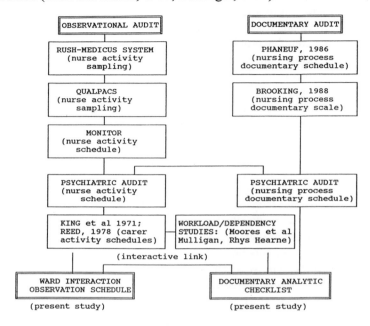

Figure 3 Developmental influences on observational and documentary measures in the present study

Characteristics of study instruments

The main innovative features and developments from current quality methods include, firstly, a DOCUMENTARY ANALYTIC CHECKLIST designed to assess the care planning records of individual patients. Based on the work of Phaneuf (1976), Hurst (1988), and Brooking (1986), this instrument employs a detailed fifty-six-item checklist that examines in depth each discrete component of individualised care as outlined within the documentation. This instrument also includes observational criteria to assess whether care planned and reflected in the documentation is actually carried out.

In order to avoid some of the criticisms described earlier, extensive developmental testing was carried out on this instrument with the help of experts within the practical field of nursing process. Similarly, validational exercises were carried out to establish objective indicators appropriate to British nursing culture and thus avoid adaptive difficulties (Brooking, 1988).

The study also utilises an innovative *ward observation schedule*, which examines the qualitative processes of forensic nursing care in detail not hitherto achieved as far as the writers are aware; and which avoids pitfalls such as artificial forcing of observations (Redfern and Norman, 1990; Oliver, 1991; Barnett and Wainwright, 1987). Current observational measures normally reflect percentage frequencies of a specific care construct or category. For example, the category "administrative behaviour" on "Jubilee Ward" may be expressed as occupying 25 per cent of nursing staff time. However, this is a global category; and precise details of the many individual behaviours occurring within the "administrative behaviour" construct are usually lost, unless the observational process is supplemented in some way (e.g., by detailed note-taking).

The observational method adopted in the present study augments this traditional quantitative approach, building upon previous work by King, Raynes and Tizard (1972) and Reed (1978); and informed by observational, dependency and workload studies of the 1970s (e.g., Moores and Grant, 1976; Moores and Moult, 1979; Mulligan, 1972, 1973; Rhys-Hearn, 1977, 1979). Whilst detailed continuous recording is a more recent method of recording activities, the problem of recording non-motor activities such as assessing and thinking, needs to be addressed. Consideration is given to the effect that self-recording has upon nurses. Rather than ticking the frequency of nursing behaviours, and assuming one of these will be observed, careful observation of *the behaviour itself* is carried out and a brief, precise description of the event recorded. This detailed record may then be retrieved at any time during subsequent analysis.

The advantage of this method is that no only can nursing behaviours be categorised qualitatively; but also the *repertoire* of behaviours occurring within the construct may be specified in fine detail and in real time. For example, the qualitative aspects of nursing care delivery may be examined by string-scanning techniques within the resultant electronic database.

These "strings" form a permanent and readily-accessed record of what actually occurred minute-by-minute during observed care sequences. It is suggested that this method may break some new ground within quality studies, by making more precise the largely unknown details of various care processes and related behaviours that occur within forensic psychiatric nursing. It is further suggested that they may possess developmental implications for quality methods within related care specialities. Although recording using radio microphones and video techniques captures detailed care processes, their "unobtrusiveness" is questionable, along with the complexity of data analysis when employing such methods. By contrast, string-scans form a much less obtrusive method by which data can be recalled instantly on any future occasion.

Regarding time-sampling techniques, the study proceeds by observing nurses for standard periods of thirty seconds, followed by thirty seconds for recording behaviours. This is carried out four consecutive times for each nurse as part of a much longer random rotational sequence in which s/he will be observed several times.

The method makes effective use of the nurse observer's time, by contrast with ten-minute and fifteen-minute sampling, which has been criticised for its wastefulness and tendency to unrepresentativeness (Balogh, 1991; West, 1991). Such criticisms cast doubt on the reliability and validity of results obtained by these methods (Smith, 1986; Barnett and Wainwright, 1987). By contrast, the use of four consecutive observations for each nurse makes more effective use of observer time and addresses the issue of picking up the pattern of constantly-changing behaviours involved in nursing activities.

Observer effects in the clarification of nursing behaviour have been a frequent problem in past studies (Tomalin, 1991; Oliver, 1991). The present study seeks to reduce these to a minimum by careful training of observers and especially by familiarising them with ward routines during a period of detailed fieldwork. Nurse observers who have formerly been part of the ward team have established themselves as reliable and valid data collectors despite the potential hazard of "halo" and Hawthorne effects.

Finally, quality instruments themselves have been criticised as lacking in validity and reliability (Smith, 1986; Redfern and Norman, 1990; Oliver, 1991; West, 1991). In the present study repeated validity and reliability checks have been carried out in a variety of contexts involving both internal and external locations during pre-pilot and pilot phases, as well as within the main investigation itself.

Research hypotheses

Research hypotheses emergent within the present study are as follows:

1   that both "mainstream" psychiatric nursing and forensic psychiatric nursing may be seen as sub-sets of a nursing culture;
2   that there are marked similarities in the pattern of operational care behaviours seen in both contexts (i.e., etic factors);
3   that there are also significant differences observable between the two contexts (i.e., emic factors);

4   that is it possible to combine both qualitative and quantitative measures and assessments to reflect the characteristics of sub-sets of nursing care;

5   that documented care reflects that which is actually given;

6   that individualised care will occur with less frequency than task-allocated types of care;

7   that *indirect* care will account for the largest proportion of nursing activities observed.

3 Method

General context and method

Special Hospitals provide treatment under secure conditions for patients suffering from a wide range of mental disorders. Rampton Hospital - one of the three English special hospitals - is managed directly by a recently established health authority, the Special Hospitals Service Authority (SHSA).   Special Hospitals treat and help almost two thousand men and women in what is intended to be a friendly and constructive atmosphere. Patients arrive in the main from the courts and remand centres, under conditions laid down in the Mental Health Act, 1983; or from local psychiatric hospitals, where they may have proved too difficult to nurse in an open setting. The nature of the patient population means that an active therapeutic policy has to be operated in a very secure setting.

Within the National Health Service Act (1977), Rampton Hospital is described as existing for the purpose of treating mentally disordered patients under conditions of special security on account of their dangerous, violent or criminal propensities. This requires the hospital effectively to combine the following general functions.

(A) CUSTODIAL: i.e., by preventing individuals from engaging in acts which could be harmful to themselves or others;

(B) PROTECTIVE: i.e., by safeguarding the rights of patients detained under the 1983 Mental

(C) Health Act;
THERAPEUTIC: i.e., by preparing them for return to less secure conditions, or to the outside community, as soon as possible.

Review of the literature

In order to establish an in-depth knowledge of nursing process, quality assurance and the current status of related research design, a review of the literature was carried out. This involved collaboration with the Staff Education Centre Library, where computer-assisted searches were organised. These facilitated further insight into the nature of these issues; established what had already been carried out in the way of related studies; and promoted insight into research designs and current thinking. A compilation of numerous journal articles and research papers, as well as related conference attendance and participation, was undertaken; and used extensively to gain relevant insights.

Limitations of the study

Although their desirability is recognised, no attempt was made in the present study to obtain external patient sub-samples drawn from a wider population of mentally handicapped people. Such investigations needs to be pursued; and will form an essential feature of further generalising studies. However, in terms of time and resources, they were beyond the scope of the present study.

It is further recognised that few, if any, empirically based studies relate to patient outcomes (Hayward, 1986). Whilst such outcome studies are also desirable, the scope of this study did not permit such measures, although it is anticipated that predictive indicators for further research of this type will emerge from it.

Location and sampling

The present study was carried out in five locations, three internal and two external to Rampton Hospital. Internal wards are coded as R1, R2 and R3 and external locations are E1, within a Mental Health Unit in Central Nottinghamshire Health Authority: and E2 within a Mental Health hospital in Wakefield Health Authority. Criteria of selection were as follows:

Care types

The three internal locations are representative of three distinctive care types within Rampton Hospital (i.e., mental illness, mental handicap and psychiatric pre-discharge areas). This criterion reflects pragmatic concerns governing the practicalities of such a study, and ensuring its utility within the primary context of forensic psychiatric nursing.

Clinical nurse specialists

They are also representative of ward which, at the time of sampling, were within the care and unifying influence of a Clinical Nurse Specialist. This was partly an opportunistic choice, since the three Clinical Nurse Specialists concerned had shown special interest in, and support for, the study. It was important to take advantage of this interest since recent police investigations had resulted in widespread staff anxiety concerning research studies. Enthusiastic Clinical Nurse Specialists would therefore play an important role in "defusing" what otherwise might be interpreted as stressful situations; and therefore make the research possible.

Training wards

The third criterion was that all five locations were designated as training wards for purposes of professional nurse education. This was considered desirable since mandatory profiling of training wards ensures, firstly, that the ward is offering varied training situations and, secondly, that the attention of clinical managers is focused on key elements of individualised care. The three internal wards are thus controlled for their degree of educational involvement.

Types of psychiatric disorder treated

The fourth criterion was that, between them, the wards should accommodate patients suffering from a variety of common psychiatric disorders and/or impairments, giving general validity to the observations carried out within each environment. This is obviously critically important where it is intended to examine the generalising properties of the research instruments as vehicles for description and analysis of nursing care for people suffering from a variety of common psychiatric disorders, both within and outside the forensic context.

Internal patient sub-samples

Patient sub-samples for the Rampton study locations were of two types. The first consisted of mentally impaired women suffering from severe to moderate degrees of mental handicap (R1). The purpose of including this sub-sample was to augment preliminary data on the nursing care of mentally impaired patients already obtained during the pilot study (Robinson, 1988).

The second type of patient sub-sample consisted of male patients accommodated in representative psychiatric wards at Rampton Hospital (R2 and R3). Patients in the selected wards are aged between twenty-eight and fifty-five years (mean age for both sub-samples 38.0 years). Arriving from courts, prison, other special hospitals, regional secure units and local psychiatric hospitals, they had been Rampton patients for periods ranging from one month to nine years (mean length of stay: R2 ward 5.9 years; R3 ward 10.3 months). Prior to their admission to Rampton all had committed one or more anti-social acts (e.g., homicide; assault; use of weapons; theft) attributable to the effects of mental illness and/or psychopathic disorder; and necessitating their compulsory detention under the provisions of the Mental Health Act, 1983.

Patients in both Rampton psychiatric sub-samples suffered from various general psychiatric disorders, including attacks of depression and/or acute anxiety (leading in some cases to suicidal or parasuicidal behaviour); social isolation; euphoric and hypomanic states, paranoid delusions and hallucinatory states, some related to substance abuse; and psychopathic personality disorders.

External patient sub-samples

The main purpose of obtaining observational data from external psychiatric wards was to augment preliminary data of this type obtained during the pilot study (Robinson, 1988). These data are of considerable importance both in validating research instruments and in assessing the generalisability of findings beyond the forensic psychiatric context of Rampton Hospital. The two external locations concerned were a psychiatric unit attached to a district general hospital in Central Nottinghamshire; and a general admission ward in a psychiatric hospital in Wakefield, West Yorkshire.

In selecting external clinical locations and sub-samples, care was taken that membership of sub-samples should reflect as far as possible the clinical characteristics observed in the relevant Rampton sub-samples: i.e., that internal and external sub-samples should be "balanced" as far as possible in clinical terms, to control for the likelihood that care behaviour of nursing staff will be affected to some extent by the nature of the clinical conditions being treated.

With the close liaison of ward staff in terms of the status of health to enable patients to be potential informants, a sub-sample of ten patients was identified for each location, giving a total patient sample of N=50.

Nursing staff sub-samples

In each ward context, observational sub-samples consisted of all nursing staff from the day shifts who were willing to participate (see Table 1). For purposes of depth interviews a random sample of ten nurses from each location was recruited, giving a total nursing staff sample of N=50.

Table 1
Skill mix of clinical nursing staff on
wards in present study (N=69)

NURSING STAFF GRADE:	RAMPTON STUDY CONTEXTS			EXTERNAL STUDY CONTEXTS	
	R1 WARD	R2 WARD	R3 WARD	E1 WARD	E2 WARD
C.N.S	1	1	1	1	1
Ward Sister/Charge Nurse	2	2	2	2	1
Registered Nurse	4	6	6	4	5
Enrolled Nurse	5	3	2	2	2
Nursing Auxiliary	5	2	2	4	3
TOTAL:	17	14	13	13	12

(C.N.S. = Clinical Nurse Specialist)

Procedure and study plan

Because of the amount of observational data to be collected within the five care settings (N= 15,000 discrete observations) it was decided to enlist the help of five nurse observers as outlined in the following sections. The general plan of the study is set out in Figure 4 (see next page).

The study extended the context of the pilot work to include five further ward locations: three internal, and two external, to Rampton Hospital. The three internal locations (R1, R2 and R3 wards) were selected as representative of mental handicap, acute psychiatric and rehabilitation services offered by Rampton Hospital; whereas the two external locations, E1 and E2 wards, were selected as analogous services in acute psychiatric and rehabilitation services provided within "mainstream" community psychiatric care.

Figure 4 outlines the logic of the work plan. Weeks 1 to 24 were devoted to an initial extended literature review in relevant aspects of nursing theory; quality care studies; research methodology; and curriculum theory (for details of review, see indicative reading list in Annexe E). In parallel with this work, detailed sampling and preliminary fieldwork in the proposed five clinical areas were carried out: three in Rampton Hospital itself; and two in additional collaborating establishments in Central Nottinghamshire and Wakefield Health Authorities. This preparatory period also saw the completion of proposed modifications to observation/interview schedules and data sheets forming the main data collection instruments for the study (see Annexes A to D).

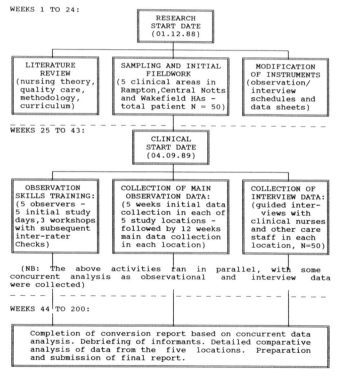

Figure 4   Overview of plan of work

Theory of observation

The methodological theories underlying this study are those of neo-realism (Russell, 1912, 1914, 1921); and of cognitive behaviourism (Meichenbaum, 1977). In terms of observational method, the researcher adopts the Russellian account of the external world as composed of sense-data. These sense-data are not physical objects, but the entities, such as pulses of sound or patches of colour, of which the observer has knowledge by acquaintance - i.e., of which s/he is immediately aware in sensation. The existence of such sense-data is fleeting and momentary; and probably does not continue after sensation has ceased. How, then, do we account for the construction of common-sense physical objects and events - the material of the observer's world?

In terms of neo-realist theory, such objects and events represent a logical construction from the different appearances that sets of sense-data present to different people. Though necessarily always unique, because perceived from a standpoint peculiar to the individual, these perceived objects and events form a system of perspectives.

Subsequent work in the psychology of perception has demonstrated that perception (including observation) is a complex skill, by no means in-built, but capable of being acquired as "a system of shared perspectives". Thus Neisser writes: "Perception - the basic cognitive activity out of which all others must emerge - is something that *mechanisms* within us do for us: it is something that *organisms* do and in particular something that *people* do" Neisser, 1976, pp 1, 9, 50). "Thus Neisser sees us as being ourselves responsible in some measure for how we see the world and as both aided and constrained by our knowledge. Just as we can be more or less skilled in our performance of our more overt activities, so we may ... be more or less skilled in our conduct of our mental activities. A skilled performer is a part of the world; he acts on it and it acts on him. Perception is also a skill ... in its continuity, in its cyclic nature, its dependence on continually modified schemata - *perceiving* is a kind of *doing*. (Shotter, 1981, p 677)."

Thus two persons whose "places" are near to each other perceive very similar perspectives; and can use the same words to denote them. Such observers can establish a correlation by means of similarity between the objects or events appearing in their immediate perspectives. This perceived congruence forms the basis of the systematic observations constituting a large part of the data of this study. Here the mode of data capture represents an innovative development from the detailed techniques initially used by King, Raynes and Tizard (1971); and by Reed (1978).

The observations consist of measurable or recordable behaviour of both nurses and patients, obtained during therapeutic and/or incidental interactions of the ward; and non-interactive behaviours, each carefully described both in qualitative and in quantitative terms. However, interpretation of these data is not left at the classic behavioural level. Instead, depth interviews are used to thrown light on the constructed social meaning of such interactions and events, as perceived both by the actors themselves and by interested others -i.e., multidisciplinary health professionals working in the hospital contexts (cf, e.g., Harre and Secord, 1972; Argyle; 1973 Meichenbaum, 1977; Wilson, 1980).

Preparation of observers

Observer curriculum

Week 25 saw the clinical start date; and was devoted to an initial intensive training block for the five nurse-observers who were involved in clinical fieldwork (see Table 2 on next page).
For purposes of monitoring nurse-observer progress during the study block, pre-and post-course questionnaires were completed (Annexes G and H). In addition guidance notes for tutors were constructed (see Annexe I). The introductory study block was also followed by an initial, closely-monitored period of four weeks observation by each observer on his/her own ward, prior to collection of main observational data on the same ward. Throughout, inter-rater reliability was monitored systematically, using the technique of dual synchronous analysis.

Field preparation of observers

During Weeks 26-30, observers were involved in preliminary data collection in their own ward contexts. This preliminary fieldwork was closely supervised by the researcher, employing frequent inter-rater reliability checks. Following this period of training in clinical fieldwork, observers proceeded to main observational data collection in each location. Synchronous data collection in the five ward locations yielded data equivalent to fifteen months of data collection by the unaided researcher. This was considered to be the optimal method, since it ensured data collection in synchrony rather than in series; produced minimal interference with the ward locations; and economised the time which clinical nurses spent in preparing for, and being involved in, active data collection.

Table 2
Curricular content of induction block
for nurse observers

TIME:	Monday 04.09.89	Tuesday 05.09.89	Wednesday 06.09.89	Thursday 07.09.89	Friday 08.09.89
09.30 - 10.30	Welcome and Overview	The Logic of Observation	Introduction to Study Instruments	Inter-rater Reliability Tests	Quality Care Forum
10.30	COFFEE				
11.00- 12.30	Methods of Qualitative analysis	Using Observation Instruments	Quality Assurance Studies	Synchronous Observation Technique	Computer Methods in quality Analysis
	LUNCH				
1.30- 2.30	Rampton Pilot Study	Observation Workshop (1)	Observation Workshop (3)	Synchronous Observation Technique (2)	Evaluation of Study Block
2.30	BREAK				
3.00- 4.00	Library Period	Observation Workshop (2)	Observation Workshop (4)	Library Period	Field-work Briefing
4.00	END OF STUDY DAY				

Rationale for employing nurse observers on their own wards

Much thought was given to the relative merits of data collection on the nurse's own or other wards. Nurse-observers working on their own wards have the considerable advantage of familiarity with the clinical context and patients concerned; and of being welcomed and trusted by patients and colleagues, to whom they are well-known and pose no threat. Conversely, some problems of objectivity, role expectations and "halo" effects beset the nurse-observer working on his/her own ward. For purposes of this study, bearing in mind time constraints and the formidable learning load which fell on nurse-observers trying to learn new clinical contexts in addition to new research techniques, the advantages of "own ward" observations were considered to outweigh any possible disadvantages, subject to monitoring provided by systematic inter-rater reliability checks.

Collection of main observational data

Ward observations were carried out at all periods of the patients' waking day, employing random rotational time-sampling technique. Scheduling of observations ensured that all periods of the day were appropriately represented in the time-bands 0730-1000; 1000-1200; 1200-1400; 1400-1600; 1600-1800; and 1800-2000 respectively. Observations were carried out in parallel with analysis of care documentation for the patient sub-samples, again carried out by the nurse-observers and checked for reliability by the researcher. Similarly, during Weeks 30-43, guided interviews with clinical nurses and patients were carried out by the researcher in each location. Some concurrent analysis of observational and interview data was carried out as the study proceeded.

Finally, during Weeks 44-200, the interim (conversion) report was completed, followed by debriefing of informants and detailed comparative analysis of data obtained from the five clinical locations: culminating in preparation of the final report.

Research instruments

Data were collected using four main research instruments initially designed and piloted during the preliminary pilot study (Robinson, 1988).

Ward observation schedule (see Annexe A)

This descriptive instrument was used for recording and evaluating a comprehensive range of nursing behaviours, including interactions occurring between nurse/nurse and nurse/patient. The innovative recording system makes it possible to obtain fine-grained details of care that can be analyzed both qualitatively and quantitatively. Resultant observations reflect the waking day of patients and permit analysis of care planned in relation to care given. The total number of observations collected in each location was 3,000 giving a total $N = 15,000$ discrete observations.

Planned and documented care needs to be seen in action as well as recorded. Currently, little is known in forensic psychiatric nursing settings as to the nature of staff/staff and staff/patient interactions, or indeed of other ward-based activities, though some relevant studies exist (cf, e.g, Cormack, 1976). This empirical approach sets out to investigate such interaction in exact detail, using methods flexible enough to offer the possibility of generalising to other ward settings. The present schedule builds on principles previously outlined in other contexts (King, Raynes, and Tizard, 1971; Reed, 1978; Davis, 1986c) to offer a description not only of elements of nursing process whenever these occur; but also of other behaviours and interactions of whatever type.

The value of this type of description becomes more apparent as more accountability is placed on the individual nurse. A paradox exists in the juxtaposition of the current need to improve patient services with current shortage of funding and poor resources. There is a growing awareness of the direct link existing between systematic individualised care and the quality of that care. If patients are to receive quality care through nursing process, suitable methods of measuring such care (i.e., suitable performance indicators) need to be introduced. Most current instruments designed for this purpose appear relatively situation-specific and perhaps not as exact as might be wished: that is, observations tend to be forced into pre-existing categories at their time of occurrence, and the character of the actual observation prematurely lost.

The Ward Observation Schedule (see Annexe A) is very simple in its basic principles, although training and skill are required to use it accurately. Behaviours are recorded on the observation sheet as briefly and accurately as possible. This provides a permanent record of behaviours made as they occur. Such behaviours are then available for categorisation on completion of each observation session. Thus the actual *nature* of the event is permanently recorded and recoverable at a later date; and the situation is not prematurely categorised with resultant loss of content.

Once the observation period is over, recorded observations can be coded either as belonging to one of eight nursing process related codes; or to one of seven non nursing process codes. Categories can be collated to give graphic or statistical profiles of the empirical nature of nursing care on the ward. Should a recorded behaviour not "fit" under any of the predetermined categories, then further consideration of its precise nature allows for the creation of another, more appropriate category. In addition to the character of such nursing behaviours, the observation sheet gives useful data on staff-patient ratios; and will highlight any patient ostensibly requiring additional care.

An additional, extremely useful feature of this instrument is its ability to distinguish, on an empirical basis, between care recorded and care delivered. By selecting an ongoing care plan and comparing the details of the proposed therapeutic intervention with care actually *delivered* to the patient, such interactions can be observed for their actual connection with the care plan: that is, the extent to which they are directed towards the achievement of manifest, care goals. *Actual* behaviours may then be evaluated against *intended* behaviours and recorded in the progress notes. This is an effective method of ascertaining the extent to which planned and documented nursing care is actually carried out.

Using the ward observation sheet (see Annexe A)

Each sheet is used for a series of four observations on *one* person only. When it is complete, another sheet is used for the next person to be observed. Each observation is made for thirty seconds, allowing a further thirty seconds for recording what is observed; and so on, until the four observations allowed for on the sheet are complete. Different sequences were tried in the pilot (Robinson, 1988); but the sequence just described appeared best to reflect the series of behaviours that nurses displayed and subsequently made effective use of observer time.

Observations are non-participant: that is, the observer was not involved in the activities of the ward team; and could concentrate on the observations only. However, should an urgent situation arise which requires the observer to intervene, then this must naturally take priority: e.g., suppose a patient has an epileptic fit, then s/he must naturally be treated for the fit as an urgent priority. The consideration of patient welfare must obviously take priority in such critical circumstances.

Observers were located in a part of the room from which each part could be observed effectively. Observations were made discreetly, and staring was avoided.

Completion of the ward observation sheet

WARD: Here the name of the ward on which the observations took place is entered.

DATE: The date on which the observations are made is recorded.

SHEET NUMBER: All sheets are numbered consecutively in the order in which they are filled in, starting with Sheet 1, then Sheet 2 and so on. Separate sequences were recorded for patient-oriented observations and staff-oriented observations.

SHEET STARTED: The time at which that specific sheet was started is entered.

SHEET COMPLETED: The time at which that specific sheet was completed is recorded.

Structure of the ward observation sheet

COLUMN 1: NS/PT (NURSE OR PATIENT): Each member of the ward nursing team was given a code by which s/he was remembered, but which did not identify him/her to others. A master list of names of nurses posted on the ward to assign individual codes was kept to assist with this; but was kept absolutely confidential.

Patient codes were also allocated and kept confidential in the same manner. For example: Fred Bloggs = A; Brian Smith = B; and so on. To avoid confusion, different code types were used for nurses and patients: that is, numbers for nurses; letters for patients. The master list was destroyed once each observer became familiar with the appropriate codes; and in any case at the end of the total observation exercise.

Codes given to members of the ward team were completely randomised to avoid possible order effects in the sequence of observations. For example, if there are six members assigned codes 1 through 6, the first observation sequence may be ordered 5,4,1,2,6,3; the second sequence may be ordered 3,1,5,6,4,2; and so on. Nursing grade was also recorded at the side of the code: e.g., CNS = clinical nurse specialist; SN = staff nurse; EN = enrolled nurse; NA = nursing auxiliary; STN = student nurse.

The code for the person being observed was then entered in Column 1, together with the appropriate nursing grade: for example, 1/SN (staff nurse); or 1/NA (nursing auxiliary).

COLUMN 2: DESCRIPTION OF BEHAVIOUR: Once the ward, date, sheet number and Column 1 sections had been completed, the observations commenced by entering the time started in the "sheet started" section.

The observer then proceeded to observe the person identified by code in Column 1. S/he was observed for thirty seconds. This was done with the aid of an unobtrusive stop-watch, or watch with second hand. Whilst observing the behaviour, the nature of any verbal interaction which occurred was also noted.

At the end of this thirty seconds, thirty seconds for recording were taken as follows:

At the end of each thirty-second observation, a concise description of the observed behaviour was written in Column 2: for example, "Helping patient to shave and giving verbal prompts on how to use the razor"; "Talking on telephone to doctor about blood pressure of John Smith".

Once the description was recorded, a circle around 0, 1 or 2 at the bottom of the box was made: 0 = indirect care; 1 = group care; 2 = individual care, whichever was appropriate to the behaviour observed and recorded.

If 0 or 1 was circled, observers proceeded to complete Columns 4, 5 and 6. Column number 3 is not completed until the end of the day's observations. This can be accurately completed then because a descriptive time capture through the description enables recording to be carried out at the end of the exercise.

If 2 was circled, then the observer went on to ring the following codes at the bottom of Column 2. These are P or N - then R, T or A: but NOT L (language) at this stage: P = patient-initiated interaction; N = nurse-initiated interaction; R = nurse rejects patient; T = nurse tolerates patient; A = nurse accepts patient.

Where language was used, one of the following codes was entered at the side of the letter L in the bottom right corner of the description of behaviour (Column 2): 1 = inaudible talk, that is the language is too quiet or the observer is too far away to hear it exactly; 2 = angry talk, that is, something said fiercely and angrily to the patient; 3 = negative control, for example, "DON'T do this, DON'T do that!"; 4 = positive control, for example, "DO this, DO that!"; 5 = programmatic talk, that is, talking the patient through a specific course of action - explaining to him what he is doing whilst he is actually doing it; 6 = explanatory talk, that is, language intended to make something clear to the patient; 7 = expressions of affection or regard, for example, gentle or considerate comments, or use of pet name.

All language usage is accompanied by *non-verbal indicators*. These consist of things like tone of voice; body posture; gestures; facial expressions, and the like. On most occasions, language and non-verbal indicators spell out the same message.

For this reason, whenever a language code is recorded the non-verbal (NV) code was inserted in the right hand side at the bottom of Column 2. This then indicates whether liking/disliking is indicated by the accompanying non-verbal behaviour of the person being observed. There are two such non-verbal codes: that is, NV2 = non-verbal expressions of anger or disliking; and NV7 = non-verbal expressions of liking or regard. For example, if speech is recorded the NV code is put in brackets after the language code, this being the non-verbal code which described the non-verbal behaviour accompanying the language: for example, 7 (NV7) where the two are "saying the same thing"; or 7 (NV2), where the talk is pleasant, but the non-verbal behaviour indicates disliking rather than liking!

On completion of these codes, Columns 4, 5 and 6 were completed as follows.

COLUMN 3: CODE: This code was entered only at the end of the day's observations, using the Ward Observation Key to decide on the correct codes (see Annexe A).

COLUMN 4: LOCATION: In this column the observer recorded the location where the observation took place: for example, dayroom (DR); ward office (WO); kitchen (KT); and so on.

COLUMN 5: NUMBER OF STAFF: In this column the number of staff present in the room or location where the observation took place was recorded.

COLUMN 6: NUMBER OF PATIENTS: In this column the number of patients present in the room or location was recorded just after the observation.

Key to ward observation codes

In order to describe observed interactions, codes were devised to categorise all observed behaviours. The key to the Ward Observation Schedule (see Annexe A) was constructed in order to facilitate easy ascription of behaviours to various codes by producing reasonably precise criteria for inclusion under each code. The codes thus created underwent some further expansion after piloting; The fifteen current care constructs represent eight nursing process (NP) and seven non-nursing process (non-NP) codes (see Tables 3 and 4, following):

Table 3
Nursing process behavioural codes

AE (ASSESSMENT EXPLICIT): that is, verbal behaviour to do with assessment of an individual patient

AI (ASSESSMENT-IMPLICIT): that is, other behaviour by which assessment of an individual patient is implied although not specifically mentioned

PE (PLANNING-EXPLICIT): that is, verbal behaviour to do with care planning for an individual patient

PI (PLANNING-IMPLICIT): that is, other behaviour by which care planning for an individual patient is *implied* but not specifically mentioned

IE (IMPLEMENTATION-EXPLICIT): that is, verbal behaviour to do with implementation of nursing care for an individual patient

II (IMPLEMENTATION-IMPLICIT): that is, other behaviour by which implementation of nursing care for an individual patient is *implied* but not specifically mentioned

EE (EVALUATION-EXPLICIT): that is, verbal behaviour to do with the evaluation of nursing care for an individual patient

EI (EVALUATION-IMPLICIT): that is, other behaviour by which the evaluation of nursing care for an individual patient is *implied* but not specifically mentioned.

Because staff-patient interactions and other ward behaviours cannot all be systematic, care constructs were developed to measure other forms, both of care given and of other duties, which could result in the observation periods recording a typical ward interactive day. The following codes represent the non-NP behavioural categories observed: (see Table 4 on next page).

Table 4
Non-NP codes

PF (PATIENT-FUNCTIONAL): that is, any general task-oriented physical care of patients which is unrelated to any individual care plan.

AS (ADMINISTRATIVE-SUPERVISORY): that is, any discussion or behaviour of a NON-PATIENT RELATED, administrative or supervisory nature.

SP (SUPERVISORY-PATIENT): that is, any patient-related discussion or interaction of a supervisory nature, but not related to an individual care plan.

PS (PATIENT-SOCIAL): that is, any general task-oriented or individual social care of patients, but unrelated to any individual care plan.

DM (DOMESTIC): that is, any non-patient-related discussion or behaviour to do with domestic issues in ward management.

MS (MISCELLANEOUS): that is, any staff discussion or behaviour which does not fit under any of the other descriptive codes.

CE (CLINICAL EDUCATION): that is, any aspects of nurse education to any members of the ward clinical team, including students.

Documentary analysis (see Annexe B)

A fifty-six-item checklist was designed to assess the calibre and completeness of recognisable care process elements in the documentation of patient care using the four discrete phases of the nursing process (assessment, care planning, implementation and evaluation). Documentary analysis data collected in each location is $N=10$, giving a total $N=50$. Documentation surrounding the nursing process is considerable: and much time and effort is required in order to deal with it sufficiently well to assess patients effectively and formulate precise, individually-tailored care plans.

Because good care planning documentation draws on many different skills, including accurate recording; effective communicative skills; and the ability to formulate realistic and achievable patient goals, documentation in the hands of disinterested or ill-prepared nurses may become a tedious exercise, resulting in anomalies such as lack of initial assessment; unrealistic goals; poor or inaccurate recording; and lack of evaluation.

The analytic checklist for documentation used in the present study was inspired by related recent work (cf, for example, Brooking, 1986); and has been specially designed to investigate separate elements of care planning under the four familiar discrete phases of the nursing process. Each of these elements would normally be regarded as part of everyday nursing care: and would be recognised as such by those using the model. The checklist of items occurring under each of the four stages of nursing process (see Annexe B) is designed to be worked through item-by-item, checking each item in turn for its existence in the documentation, and scoring it accordingly as follows (see Table 5 on next page).

All nursing records in relation to each patient, with special reference to his care plan(s) and treatment record(s), were examined. Taking each checklist item in turn, each was assessed for its presence against the related documentation and scored using the criteria in Table 5.

In relation to the care plans and other nursing process documents for each patient, each was allocated a score ranging from zero (no record) to 3 (a clear, detailed and informative record). When completed, the checklist was analysed for low-scoring areas, relating either to individuals or to groups of patients. This results in a precise description of the characteristics of documented care. Investigation of documented care is important since without such records little useful evaluation can be carried out regarding patient outcomes; and no form of continuity can be offered either within or between shifts.

Table 5
Documentary analysis - criteria for
scoring checklist items

NO RECORD (NR)	indicates that the item cannot be found in any of the documents examined (i.e., NO ATTEMPT MADE - SCORE O)
PARTIAL RECORD (PR)	indicates that a relatively brief and uninformative mention of the item can be found. EXAMPLE FOR ITEM 6: "Rather anxious this morning". (i.e., SLIGHT ATTEMPT MADE - SCORE 1)
INCOMPLETE RECORD (IR)	indicates that, although an appreciable attempt has been made, the item is recorded in an unclear or ambiguous manner. EXAMPLE FOR ITEM 6: "Rather anxious this morning due to family problems". (i.e., FAIR ATTEMPT MADE - SCORE 2)
COMPLETE RECORD (CR)	indicates that a clear, detailed and informative mention of the item can be found. EXAMPLE FOR ITEM 6: "Rather anxious this morning in anticipating a visit from his parents. This anxiety is apparently due to his concern about his brother's drug problem. Bill fears that it is killing him. Reassured that his brother is receiving treatment. After the visit, Bill became more like his normal self again". (i.e., GOOD ATTEMPT MADE - SCORE 3)

Patient guided interview schedule (see Annexe C)

This semi-structured or guided interview schedule was used to gain insights into patients' perceptions of, and attitudes towards, nursing care received in a specific care environment. Interviews in each location numbered N=10, giving a total patient sample of N=40. Due to the severe handicap of patients within R1 ward, sampling was abandoned on this ward due to communication problems.

Few, if any, studies in the forensic psychiatric nursing field have invited patients to express their perceptions of their care (SHSA, 1991). From the outset, the present study recognised the potential importance of such views; and the desirability of involving patients in planning their own nursing care.

There is an obvious caveat to be entered concerning the degree of psychiatric impairment which a patient may be experiencing at the time of care planning; with its potential for producing unreliable data. This schedule is designed to approach individual patients in an understandable, friendly and non-threatening way, building on much personal contact and familiarity with individual patients deliberately fostered as a critical part of the "groundwork" from the start of the study. The importance of the researcher/patient relationship in acquiring valid data cannot be overstressed in using this schedule.

Section A: employment and recreational interests

This consists of four questions and probes designed to gain an insight into the patient's background, employment and interests before arriving at Rampton Hospital; and so on, through to present recreational interests. These were felt to be of special interest, not only to give an insight into the individual whom the researcher is dealing with; but more specifically as a means of setting the patient at ease in the interview situation; and also of ascertaining to what degree the patient's interests are shared with staff or with other patients.

Section B: patient's perceptions of care

This consists of six questions and probes directed at the patient's perceptions of, and involvement with planning of, his own nursing care. The quality of nurse/patient relationships is an important feature of any nursing environment; therefore it was considered appropriate to examine this area. Since the patient should ideally be involved in planning his own care, it was necessary to assess each patient's perceptions, both of his care needs and of care actually received, in order to evaluate the involvement as perceived by individual patients.

In addition, it was considered useful to gain an insight into the current care plan, and related care given by nurses, as seen by the patient. Because of the secure Rampton environment, patients are widely held to view the hospital as a prison. During the course of the study useful data were gathered regarding this supposed "penal" view of Rampton care.

Section C: family and other outside contacts

Perceived isolation can exert a direct effect upon responses to therapy. Due to limited visiting and Rampton's nationwide catchment, it was considered useful to establish to what extent patient contacts with relatives and friends were maintained; and whether or not patients thought that relatives could help them in any specific way.

Nurse interview schedule (see Annexe D)

This schedule is very similar in structure and purpose to the patient guided interview schedule, but is in greater depth and geared towards professional issues. Interviews in each location numbered N=10, giving a total nursing staff sample of N=50.

For the purposes of investigating the nurses' perceptions of, and attitudes towards, the nursing process, a semi-structured interview schedule was designed. This originally took the form of unstructured questions to elicit information concerning nursing process. During the design phase experienced and knowledgeable informants from general, psychiatric and mental handicap fields of nursing were invited to respond to unstructured questions.

Resultant data were recorded on audiotape and analysed for content areas relating to the nursing process. The resultant schedule which gradually emerged consisted of a semi-structured interview involving four main sections. Each section dealt with a main area of inquiry, with further questions and probes under each of the four main sections.

Section A: background information

This consists of four questions and probes designed to give an insight into the background, education and qualifications acquired by the informant up to the time of entering nursing. These data would, it was anticipated, reveal any influences both in practical and attitudinal approaches to nursing care, as seen by people who have gained other skills before entering nursing; and help to assess whether or not their attitudes differed from those of direct entrants to nursing.

Section B: professional background and perceived role

This consists of ten questions and probes designed to investigate the informant's previous experience in nursing through to his present post. It was felt important to look at how much education nurses had received, and in what areas it had been undertaken. This was especially important as regards the evolution of the nursing process at Rampton Hospital, to gain an insight into the type and amount of resources channelled to nurses to help them come to terms with this important concept.

Of equal importance was the need to look at future in-service education requirements as perceived by the nurses themselves; and at the skills which nurses felt they could currently contribute towards patient care; their perceptions of current and future involvement with patients; and their future career development. This it was felt would then give a reasonably accurate account of nursing resources and types of preferred involvement with patients, as well as highlighting special skills and interests of the nursing staff concerned.

Section C: ward/unit care planning and communication

This consists of thirteen questions and probes designed to investigate nurses' attitudes to, and perceptions of, patient needs in terms of individual requirements. It was considered important to establish whether or not individual patients were being catered for through the systematic concept of nursing process; and to evaluate to what extent nurses involved patients in formulating care plans; whether or not care planning was directly or indirectly related to the patient's needs on, or reasons for, admission; and how nursing staff ensured patients received effective nursing care.

Additionally, it was decided to ascertain whether or not nurses felt that individual care plans actually helped patients to solve their problems; and whether or not nurses felt that individual care plans actually helped patients to solve their problems; and how realistic they felt the aims to be. Patients frequently remain uninvolved in care planning ostensibly due to their related problems. In order to investigate current patient involvement, questions concerning both patient awareness of their care, and patient involvement in care planning were built into the schedule.

By these means it was hoped to assess the views of the nurses on patient involvement; and to what extent nurses involved individual patients when planning their nursing care. Ideally, care planning should be pursued on a multidisciplinary basis; and in order to establish to what extent care plans were communicated to other disciplines, and to what extent their members were involved in the construction of individual care plans, this section also includes questions relating to such multidisciplinary involvement, and related communication of care plans as perceived by the ward nursing team.

Section D: general perceptions of the nursing process

This consists of sixteen questions and probes relating to nurses' attitudes to, and perceptions of, the nursing process, from its first appearance at Rampton Hospital up to and including, its present operational status. To gain an insight into the nurses' knowledge of the concept, it was important to establish their own definition(s) of the model; their reactions to it when first implemented; and their perceptions of the advantages and disadvantages of the problem-solving approach.

Whilst noting that differences in capacity to recall necessarily affected the quality of data obtained from the nurses, it was considered important to investigate, as far as possible, their initial perceptions; their colleagues' perceptions; and their impressions of the preparation for change which they received when the nursing process was first introduced; including related courses and continuing education. Planning for change is an important concept; its strategies require much thoughtful preparation; and it was hoped that these data would give more insight into the actual impact of change strategies adopted by management when introducing this new concept to the Rampton workforce.

Additionally, it is necessary to gain certain skills, such as communication skills, in order to carry out the nursing process effectively. It was, therefore, important to look both at what nurses actually received in terms of skills preparation; and at what they felt was lacking, or still required. Not only was it important to see how nurses described the concept of the nursing process -it was equally important to gain an insight into their problem-solving approaches, which are implicit in the model, to discover whether or not nurses were utilising a genuinely systematic approach to care.

Although in the initial stages a nursing process co-ordinator was appointed to monitor care planning throughout Rampton Hospital, this role had been discontinued by the time of the study. It was therefore important to obtain nurses' perceptions of the value or otherwise of such support, in order to establish its likely impact as a change strategy.

Section E: monitoring care

This section consists of four questions and probes and is the main addition following the pilot (Robinson, 1988). This section deals with monitoring care, especially the nursing process. Similarly it looks at such issues as how nurses can improve care for patients; and whether or not care should be monitored. Finally, even though patients very rarely came into contact with night nursing staff, it was still important to gain their views on the impact of care planning during the night period, in order to assess the potential value of night shift care plans to the hospital as a whole.

Main data collection

Following training of nurse observers, main runs of data were collected. The data collected were both quantitative and qualitative in nature and included:

i   qualitative accounts of staff and patient attitudes and perceptions;
ii   quantitative and qualitative accounts of observational and documentary data.

Observational data

Times when care plan entries within the documentation were least in use were noted. Care plans and related documentation were taken to a quiet area within each location for assessment following permission of the ward sister/charge nurse. Individual care plans were subjected to detailed analysis by means of the documentary analysis (see Annexe B). Each checklist item was checked for its presence or absence in the documentation of planned care. The checklist was worked through systematically, each item receiving an appropriate score on the four-point scale. No problems were encountered, with data collection running smoothly.

Using non-participant, random rotational time-sampling techniques, main observations were carried out recording data directly onto the ward observation schedule (see Annexe A). This was done by planning data collection sequences so that observations covered all times of day and days of the week, over a period of twelve months. These data could then be examined for representativeness of a typical patient waking day; as well as for future cut-off points for data collection (see Figure 5). Observationally sequences were kept to a maximum period of four hours, inclusive of brief rest periods, to avoid fatigue and loss of vigilance on the part of nurse observers.

Each participant was observed for thirty seconds; and each observation recorded as briefly and accurately as possible during a further thirty-second period. Observation then started again until four consecutive observations were carried out, each followed by a thirty-second recording interval. After the complete rotational sample had been observed, a ten-minute rest period was taken before commencing the next randomised sequence.

Observations appeared to proceed very well; and observers encountered no major problems. Initial data were examined for any possible Hawthorne effects; but, little contamination could be found, with participants settling down to their normal routine after the first few minutes of observation. It is considered that this result was mainly due to the extensive fieldwork and familiarisation exercises carried out prior to the data collection phase; and to the acceptability and trustworthiness of the nurse observers within the perceptions of members of the various ward teams.

Interview data

Interview data were collected using the semi-structured interview schedules (see Annexes C and D) within an informal, non-threatening and familiar setting in the ward environment. Interviews were conducted and recorded using a small, inconspicuous audiotape recorder. Each informant was made at ease before the interview by general discussion of current topics; including a brief oral introduction to the study. No methodological problems were encountered with the collection of interview data; and all informants appeared quite relaxed and responsive, with no patient informants deciding to withdraw.

In arranging and conducting interviews for all informants, major factors likely to influence the validity and reliability of the interviews were borne in mind. These included appropriate structuring and vocabulary in the interview schedules; piloting and approvals; use of non-leading questions and probes; logic of the questioning sequence; attention to perceptual, visual and vocal cues from informants; avoidance of multiple or catch-all questions; cultivation of sensitivity, empathy, adaptability and self-awareness on the part of the interviewer; and tolerance and use of silence in interviews (see for example Brenner, 1985; Powney and Watts, 1987).

Interviews were arranged to take place at periods when the ward was least busy: and were conducted in a relatively quiet location, removed from interruptions by telephone or other staff or patients. In many cases this location was a small interview room situated within the ward.

Interviews were audiotaped using a Tandy Realistic CTR-75 voice-actuated cassette tape recorder with DC 6-volt cells (AA x 4) (catalogue number 14-800), linked to a Tandy Realistic ultra-thin omnidirectional microphone (catalogue number 33-1089). Interviews were recorded onto TDK DC90 cassette tapes for permanent storage. Use of the above equipment was found to be especially satisfactory, since the tape recorder is small and non-threatening; and the microphone ensured pickup of both direct and reflected signals at the same time, reducing feedback and eliminating interference. This strategy made it possible to record excellent quality cassettes of each interview in a non-threatening environment.

The use of the recording equipment generally was well-accepted; and it did not appear to restrict informants in their discussion. Each informant was, however, given the option either to be audiotaped or have his/her responses recorded by hand. Of the study sample, twenty informants preferred not to be audiotaped. These were all patients. Some informants requested to hear the audiotapes to evaluate their performance once the data had been transcribed and analysed. Close contact was maintained with patients in all locations to maintain rapport and confidence before the guided interviews. Contact was also maintained with ward managers and staff regarding each patient's condition both before and during interviews, to avoid subjecting anyone to undue anxiety.

Reliability and validity

Regular visits were made by the researcher to each ward, both for purposes of mentoring and to obtain inter-rater reliability measures. Inter-rater reliabilities for the nurse observers were as follows:

R1 WARD: 0.82, 0.84, 0.81, 0.86 (mean reliability 0.83);
R2 WARD: 0.82, 0.84, 0.84, 0.86 (mean reliability 0.85);
R3 WARD: 0.86, 0.84, 0.84, 0.86 (mean reliability 0.85);
E1 WARD: 0.86, 0.88, 0.86, 0.86 (mean reliability 0.86);
E2 WARD: 0.83, 0.83, 0.86, 0.85 (mean reliability 0.84);

The mean inter-rater reliability for all nurse observers was 0.84. Similarly, reliability studies of the documentary analyses showed a mean reliability coefficient of 0.83 with no reliabilities falling below 0.78. Reliability studies of interview data as revealed by content analysis and the submission of transcriptions to informants for verification have shown a high level of consistency in the data concerned.

At the time when observational data were being collected on E1 Ward, the research nurse was completing a ward audit using Psychiatric Audit (Hurst and Howard, 1989). Whilst the majority of data collected within this audit is different in nature from that of the present study, it was possible to compare the nursing behaviours. Psychiatric Audit data and data obtained during this study were compared; and results were congruent within 3 per cent. This is to some degree illustrative of the reliability of the present study data, and an indicator of its cross-validational status.

Random interviews were selected and selected questions were asked by two interviewers on separate occasions (that is, by the researcher and another interviewer). Results were highly congruent. Using key words and phrases from each interview, comparisons were made and an agreement of 81 per cent was established. Similarly, audiotape transcriptions were translated on a random basis by the researcher and assistant and results compared. Again close themes and similarities were obtained. Results showed an 84 per cent agreement. Random transcriptions were also taken back to informants and the informant asked if the transcription reflected what he had said. No informants reflected any misinterpretation, although two felt they would now like to make additional comments.

Initial validity studies were pursued by submitting the instruments to a panel of experts for their comments on both face and content validity. The panel of experts consisted of experienced researchers, experts in nursing process and in quality care studies. Few negative comments were made; and suggested modifications were carried out at an early stage. Content validity and construct validity on all instruments were established and rechecked at regular intervals during pre-pilot and pilot phases. In addition, regular dissemination of the study findings, at a variety of in-house seminars and conferences at both national and international level, enabled further extended validation (see section on modifications made following the pilot study).

Validity sample

The sample involved was as follows:

Table 6
Validity sample

Academic Nurse Researchers	4	Academic Supervisors	2
Nursing Process Coordinators	3	Quality Expert	1
Nurse Educators	4	Quality Managers	8
Senior Nurse Managers	4	Patients	4
Ward-based Nurses	6		
TOTAL N: 36			

Subsequently these studies were extended by the submission of transcripts to informants for qualitative validation.

Ethical implications

Each informant (total N=119) received a personal invitation to participate in the study, together with a brief, clear written description of the nature of the exercise. From the outset, it was made clear that all participation was voluntary; that all informants had the right to refuse to participate; and that, should they elect to participate, they had the further right to abandon the exercise at any time should they so wish.

Preservation of confidentiality was stressed; along with procedures for the safe-keeping of data records. It was also made clear that, should any direct quotation be considered necessary within the interim or final reports, permission from the individual(s) concerned would be sought. Because computers were being used to store data, advice was sought from the local data protection manager, and subsequent registration gained in accordance with the requirements of the Data Protection Act, 1986.

In order to safeguard patients compulsorily detained under the provisions of the 1983 Mental Health Act, written permission for their participation from their Responsible Medical Officers and from the ward team were obtained, in addition to their own consent. As with all research carried out at Rampton Hospital, a proposal was put before the hospital Ethics Committee, to ensure that all ethical considerations were being appropriately met.

Data analysis

Analysis of interview data

In order to analyse the interview data, the audiotape containing each informant's data was transcribed onto separate data sheets, employing the main section headings of the interview schedule (Robinson, 1988). These were successfully used in the pilot and were felt accurately to represent nurse and patient interview data. By use of content-analytic techniques (Polit and Hungler, 1989) themes and trends existing within the data were identified and described. These were categorised within the main headings along with frequencies of staff grade. Similarities existing within the discrete data sets were allowed to emerge, rather than forcing certain types of data into pre-determined categories. Frequencies of similarities were recorded, supported by typical descriptive quotations summarising collective views. It was felt important that words from the "horse's mouth" were used accurately to portray the area discussed.

The documentary data in patient care plans were analysed by examining the checklist item scores for low-scoring areas; and by content analysis of the supporting descriptive data.

In order to analyse the main observational data, a specially-designed database was prepared using the current version of Masterfile PC. Here each of the discrete data areas present in the ward observation schedule was built into the database as a data input field. By entering each data item from the ward observation schedule it was then possible to carry out both quantitative and qualitative analysis, using the powerful and sophisticated calculations and comparisons resident within the database. This was done by using string-scanning techniques which enable the user to identify and count key words or phrases. As with other analysis, these can subsequently be combined and compared with any of the other data field inputs. This has considerably facilitated fast and reliable analysis and comparison of ward observation data.

At this stage statistical routines have been restricted, since the main focus of these early studies is more properly qualitative and descriptive. The statistical tests which have been included will serve as examples of the types of statistical analysis which will become increasingly necessary and appropriate in future studies, as appropriate data accumulates.

Statistical analysis using Spearman's rank order correlation test was carried out on selected data sets. This was carried out to determine the relationship between internal and external study locations. The statistical analysis carried out offers further support for frequency and descriptive accounts of study trends. Further data from internal and external locations are required from future studies in order to make additional comparisons.

Modifications following pilot study

Modifications to the instruments following the pilot study included the following amendments:

1. The Ward Observation Schedule received an additional coding category CE (clinical education). The patient- or nurse-initiated interaction codes, the rejection, toleration and acceptance (RTA) codes, language (L) and non-verbal (NV) codes were included following identification of more detailed empirical data during pilot observations. In addition responses to various comments made during validation were built in as appropriate.

2. The Documentary Analysis was modified, with an additional, more in-depth scoring criterion consisting of a scale of 0 to 3 rather than 0 to 2, since it was felt that the existing scoring was too narrow. Some checklist items were slightly re-worded and an additional checklist item was added, making a total of 56 items.

3. The Patient Interview Schedule received minor alterations to terminology, ensuring that there were standardised terms for both internal and external locations.

4. The Nurse Interview Schedule also received minor amendments to terminology; a question was added to Section C (C13); and an additional section (Section D); with one additional question in Section E (E2).

4 Observational findings

Quantitative and qualitative analysis

One of the main features of this study has been the descriptive style of recording. This has been one of the key innovative aspects of observational data capture and analysis. Whilst quantitative results are important, the ability also to interrogate them for qualitative detail is extremely important. For example, if we know that a certain behaviour is happening for 20 per cent of the time, what does 20 per cent actually mean? What are the behaviours and characteristics that actually make this up?

The caring process used by nurses involves an extremely complicated process of interactions. These interactions are far ranging and extremely varied. Nurses continue to interact in and out of a range of behaviours during one interaction. For example, a nurse may start by talking to a patient about a programme of dressing. Then she may assist her with actually getting dressed. Whilst these are two very related interactions about assisting a patient to get dressed, they are clearly two different behaviours.

Through observed "time capsules" of care it is possible to separate these distinct and different behaviours. Only when we have these precise details of care will we be able to understand the true nature of the process of nursing within a given culture. Similarly, it is interpreting these precise details that enables us to alter and manipulate care practice. Therefore this chapter will set out to examine the quantitative aspects in relation also to qualitative detail, where certain anomalies or deficits exist.

Development of electronic database for analysis

Data obtained by means of the ward observation interaction schedule were analyzed using a specially designed computerised database. Special programming of Masterfile PC database to receive data transferred from the observation sheet was undertaken and successfully completed.

Utilisation of the database facilitates fast access to, and analysis of, observational data. Although currently data are input and relevant comparisons performed manually, further development will enable even faster data access using specially programmed macros (i.e., automations of data comparison that can be sent to the printer output at the stroke of a key). These developments are outlined in the following section, along with additional recent data findings.

Each data field can be compared with any other field, or with multiple fields, offering many permutations for fine-grained analysis of both quantitative and qualitative data types. Similarly, string-scans to search out key words are a central feature; and extremely important when grouping certain interactions through content analysis. At the time of writing, more than 190 possible comparisons have been identified.

Observational data types

These include, for example, permutations of the following data types (see Figure 5):

Table 7
Observational data types

(a)	Nursing process behaviours
(b)	Non-Nursing process behaviours
(c)	Grades of staff
(d)	Days of the week
(e)	Times of day
(f)	Direct, group and indirect types of care
(g)	Types of language used
(h)	Rejecting, tolerating and accepting responses
(i)	Non-verbal responses
(j)	Nurse-initiated or patient-initiated responses
(k)	String-scans of descriptive data
(l)	Staff/patient ratios

Representativeness of observational data

Each data set was examined at five successive cumulative frequencies of 600 observations, through to the total observations collected (N=3000), to determine how many observations would constitute a "representative" figure, accurately picturing a typical waking day for patients. A waking day for patients in this instance means from their rising in the morning to retiring to bed in the evening (a time span of approximately 0730 hours to 2100 hours).

There arrives a time when data collected become "representative" in this sense. It may then be argued that further data-collection in excess of the "representative" frequencies does not serve a really useful purpose; especially when observational data collection is both time-consuming and observer-intensive. These comparisons would also yield useful data "cut-offs" on which to base future data collection strategies allowing for optimal data collection in future studies.

Figure 5 compares the pattern of observations at successive cumulative frequencies of +600, ranging from f=600 through to f=3000. As can be seen from the data, there appears to be a "critical" frequency of approximately 600-1000 observations, which represent a typical patient waking day. There appears little difference in the proportionality of behaviours occurring from 600 to 3000 observations. This in turn suggests a possible future practical "cut-off" for observational data collection. This cut-off point would, therefore, be considered "typical" at around 600-1000 observations.

However, in order to present an adequately balanced picture, a minimum frequency of some 2400 observations would be required from any ward context. In this case a complete picture relates to a detailed observational analysis representing a full seven days, including time-of-day and day-of-week analysis. The collection and monitoring of large amounts of data such as these are vital if one is reliably to represent ward activities at a level which is realistic. The key to the observation codes for Figures 5 and 6 can be found in Table 8.

Similarly, the data were examined to establish the variance of observations between the highest peak and lowest trough. Analysis revealed that, within the category of "administrative supervisory" behaviour, a frequency variation of plus-minus 1.5 per cent occurred. In other behavioral categories the frequency variation was as follows: "patient functional", plus-minus 1.5 per cent; "patient social", plus-minus 2 per cent; "nursing process" activities, plus-minus 1.5 per cent; "miscellaneous", plus-minus 2 per cent; "clinical education", plus-minus 1.5 per cent; and "domestic", plus minus 0.5 per cent.

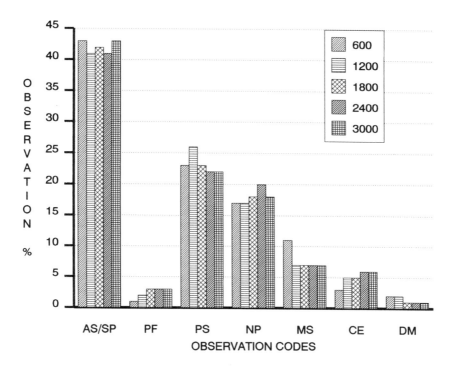

Figure 5 Comparative patterns of ward observations (N=600-3000)

Whilst there are slight peaks and troughs in the behaviours there appears to be one rather higher frequency variation in behaviour type - the increase in nursing process behaviours observed at f = 1800 - which may be accounted for by a specific intervention. This effect it is thought may be due to the impact of a clinical teaching package on the nursing process activities recorded during this period. This may account for the increase in frequency from 17 per cent at f=600 and f=1200 to 20 per cent at f=2400.

The teaching package ran concurrently during this period and was completed without further follow-up after this time. There is a decrease in frequency of observed nursing process behaviours after this period; and it is thought that the lack of follow-up, or a "settling down" effect, may account for the slight decrease in NP behaviour at f=3000. A further causal factor may be the increased turnover of some ward-based staff which also occurred at that time.

Table 8
Key to observation codes

AS (administrative-supervisory) = non-patient-related discussion or behaviour of an administrative or supervisory nature. Examples include paperwork; answering the telephone; checking stocks or giving instructions.

SP (supervisory-patient) = patient-related discussion or interaction of a supervisory nature. Examples include supervising toileting or bathing; counselling or giving instructions to patients; advising or discussing care.

PS (patient-social) = task-oriented social care of patients unrelated to individual care plans. Examples include saying good morning/goodbye to patients; playing games with, or watching television with, patients.

PF (patient-functional) = general task-oriented physical care of patients, unrelated to individual care plans. Examples include helping patients to get up or to walk; wiping bottoms or noses; washing or drying of patients.

NP (nursing process) = verbal or non-verbal interactions to do with any of the stages of care planning: that is, assessment care planning; implementation and evaluation. Examples include filling in assessment forms; giving care to patients as prescribed in individual care plans; and evaluating care.

DM (domestic) = non-patient-related discussion or behaviour to do with domestic issues in ward management. Examples include cleaning or polishing floors; washing objects; or clearing away after play sessions.

MS (miscellaneous) = examples of staff discussion or behaviour which do not fit under any of the other descriptive codes; and in which no recognisable nursing element can be found. Examples include chit-chat between staff; eating or drinking; staff in toilet or talking to researcher.

CE (clinical education) = This code refers to all aspects of nurse education to all members of the clinical team. Examples include discussions of ward procedures, updating, carrying out procedures as part of nurse training, lectures or seminars by the ward team or tutors.

Observational comparisons

Observational findings for both internal and external wards were examined and are presented in Figure 6.

Whilst there is only a small variance of observations presented in Figure 5, it is refreshing to see within Figure 6 that the observation schedule is capable of picking up the constant changes occurring in the nursing environment and thus reflecting the subtle differences in frequency of care delivery.

These changes clearly reflect actual differences between each ward; and especially between internal and external locations. As can be seen there are similarities in most areas. Broad similarities exist within the administrative and supervisory-patient (AS and SP) categories (range 21-49 per cent); patient social (PS) (range 13-28 per cent); nursing process (NP) (range 11-20 per cent); miscellaneous (MS) (range 7-17 per cent); clinical education (CE) (range 3-9 per cent); patient functional (PF) (range 3.14 per cent); and domestic (DM) (range 2-5 per cent).

The data within figure 6 were subject to statistical analysis using Spearman's rank order correlation test to determine the relationship between two data sets, i.e. two wards. It is drawn to the reader's attention at this point that in general similarities are left to interpretation through descriptive and frequency analysis presented within the figures, although examples of further statistical routines are given later.

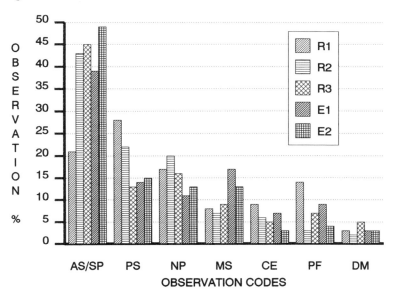

Figure 6 Inter-ward observational comparisons

The data compared are the seven care constructs, i.e., administration/patient supervision; patient-functional; patient-social; nursing process; miscellaneous; clinical education and domestic categories. Using this routine the following comparisons were made:

Wards R1 and R3, $p < 0.025$ one-tailed; $p < 0.05$ two-tailed; t-ratio=2.606; D.F $= 5$ and rho $= 0.759$.

Wards R2 and R3, $p < 0.025$ one-tailed; $p < 0.05$ two-tailed; t-ratio $= 3.879$; D.F $= 5$ and rho $= 0.866$.

Wards R3 and E1, $p < 0.025$ one-tailed; $p < 0.05$ two-tailed; t-ratio $= 3.581$; D.F $= 5$ and rho $= 0.848$.

Wards R3 and E2, $p < 0.05$ one-tailed; $p < 0.01$ two-tailed; t-ratio $= 6.024$; D.F $= 5$ and rho $= 0.938$.

These results show highly significant relationships between both internal and external data sets, which further support the graphical interpretation presented in figure 6.

It is now worth taking a closer look at these broad similarities; and attempting to draw certain inferences. First, taking the two external locations (E1 and E2 wards) there is a similar trend within both data sets.

Qualitative analysis

Qualitative analysis reveals some idiosyncratic feature of each of these wards which account for the variance within the broad themes. The high AS frequencies occurring in E2 ward clearly reflected nurses' practice of supervising patients "from the armchair" rather than being more therapeutically interactive, for example through one-to-one or group programmes. There was a similarly high frequency of PS behaviours, arising due to a member of staff who saw his role as administrator rather than as nurse.

By contrast, E1 ward AS frequencies were considerably less, due to a more eclectic care approach that saw a variety of multidisciplinary staff involved within the ward, each taking his or her responsibility for administration rather than passing this task to nursing staff. However, a higher frequency of miscellaneous behaviours for this ward meant that there was a higher ratio of interactive patient care on E2 ward. A caveat is that, although nurses on E1 ward spent much of the miscellaneous time in making drinks for themselves, they were often involved in conversation with patients during this period; and this in itself could be classed as "therapeutic" behaviour.

Regarding the three internal Rampton locations (R1, R2 and R3), R2 and R3 were very similar in their broad activities. However, R1 does stand out as being somewhat different. Firstly, it is a ward for female patients; and secondly, it accommodates patients suffering from a severe mental impairment. Clearly this ward reflects a much lower frequency of AS behaviours; and is compensated by much higher frequencies of PS and PF behavioural types. Patients with severe mental impairment require considerable input on a one-to-one basis.

Qualitative analysis reveals the nature of the interactions occurring with severely mentally impaired patients. These were particularly frequent within PF categories, where nurses were very much involved with the physical side of caring. These interactions accounted for behaviours such as helping patients to dress; assisting with personal hygiene; and assisting with meals. The PS category reflected much love and affection shown to patients by staff through verbal interactions and in particular through patients hugging and cuddling staff and vice versa.

The remaining two internal wards (R2 and R3) again appear very similar, with the main difference appearing in the PS category. R1 is an admission ward whilst R2 ward is a pre-discharge area. The PS activities as reflected by content and descriptive analysis show patients being much more involved with nursing staff in the latter context. This is reflected in a variety of interactions which include in particular general conversation about daily and life events; but particularly in socialisation through interactions, where staff form effective and lasting relationships with patients through game playing. These activity include games such as dominoes, cards and snooker. PF categories also reflect a differing scenario of events between the two wards. There is a difference here in that the R3 admission ward clearly reflects staff doing things for patients because of security and safety reasons, since newly-admitted patients are often an unknown quantity until assessments and relationships have been established. In the case of R2, patients are either ready or being prepared for discharge; and the lower frequencies of PF behaviours here reflect less dependency of patients on staff, as well as much higher levels of mutual trust.

In this section some of the qualitative detail that makes different settings vary from each other has been briefly described; and an illustration offered of how it is possible to explain certain differences through qualitative analysis. Without descriptive evidence it would be very difficult indeed to attempt explanation of such similarities or differences. In order to develop this discussion, the various care processes taking place in one ward will now be discussed in more detail.

R3 ward was chosen because the quantitative findings are "middle of the road". In order to present these details an account of the quantitative results is given followed by descriptive accounts of the content of each category. Figure 7 shows the analysis of total ward observations (f=3000) for R3. The key to codes is in Table 7.

As can be seen from Figure 7 AS (administrative supervisory) and SP (supervisory patient) behaviours, which are similar in nature, account for 45 per cent of observations. This is followed by a sharp decline in frequency to NP (nursing process) behaviours, which account for 16 per cent of observations. There is a further decline in frequency to PS (patient-social) behaviours which account for 13 per cent of observations; with MS (miscellaneous) behaviours account for 9 per cent of observations. The decline in frequency continues with PF (patient-functional) behaviours accounting for 7 per cent; CE (clinical education) behaviours for 5 per cent; and finally DM (domestic) behaviours for 5 per cent of observations.

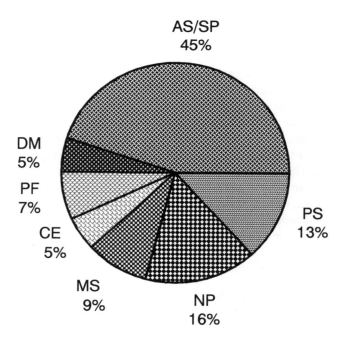

Figure 7 Total ward observations (Ward R3, N = 3000)

The two administrative behavioural categories (AS, SP) are similar in nature and have been retained together for comparative purposes with the pilot data. However, when separating them they account for administrative (AS) 20 per cent and supervision of patients (SP) 25 per cent of observed behaviours.

Within the administrative category of care the charge nurse was clearly the team member who was most involved. Behaviours and tasks with which the charge nurse was involved with were mainly administrative in nature. For example, there was considerable time spent in filling-in nursing notes; report writing in patients' files; completing monthly reports and staff rotas; opening mail and responding to requests for information. Considerable time was also spent answering the telephone. This was mostly patient related but often contained personal messages and enquiries for other team members.

Similarly, considerable time was spent in dealing with visitors to the ward for clinical purposes; such as updating senior managers and dealing with responsible medical officers (RMOs) and other medical personnel. In addition there were periods when external visitors came to the ward on planned visits which sometimes took considerable time away from ward matters.

Finally, the supervision of staff, along with preparing staffing duty rotas, was a key role of the charge nurse. Rarely observed was any delegation and planning of nursing care, involving allocation of key nurses to specific patients. Regarding the supervision of patients the charge nurse, whilst having some contact (usually through the patient coming to him), rarely supervised patients outside the office context.

It is quite clear that the charge nurse, though a highly trained team member, spends considerable amounts of his time in less patient-involved activities that perhaps a ward clerk or more junior staff might become involved in. Reluctant to leave the office, the charge nurse's skills are not utilised to the full.

Little difference if any could be found between the administrative role of the charge nurse and that of the clinical nurse specialist, since both appeared to be mainly involved in documentation of various kinds, including staffing and holiday rotas and completing nursing notes. Perhaps the only difference is that of administrative communications to nursing staff, particularly the domain of the charge nurse. Clearly the person in charge emphasised his role as resource manager to the exclusion of his role as clinician.

Staff nurses also spent considerable amounts of time in AS activities, although there were differences between their activity pattern and that of the charge nurse. Much time was spent in reading nursing notes, such as the daily report book; and in their completion at the end of the day. Similarly, staff nurses sorted mail and were partially involved in helping to construct staff duty rotas.

Telephone answering was another key area, as was preparation and completion of drug charts and ordering of drugs and various commodities. Whilst not as involved in AS activities as the charge nurse, staff nurses appeared distinctly reluctant to leave the ward office at times. This possibly indicates role uncertainty, with the ward routine taking them along, rather than any planned or coordinated schedule of patient care. Similarly the ward office was sometimes seen as a meeting point for nurses to sometimes "hang out" and chat about personal issues.

Enrolled nurses appear to play a rather different role within the administrative category. Interactions and behaviours appear to be that of delegated duties, or duties that perhaps no one else wants at the time. The enrolled nurse seems to have little influence within the ward office scenario, as tasks tend to be delegated to them by the charge nurse and staff nurses. It appears almost as if they do not want enrolled nurses interfering to any great extent in what is seen as their role.

However enrolled nurses are involved in some documentation completion such as maintaining seclusion records; writing on the patients' information board; writing some day reports in the nursing notes; and completing requisition forms on behalf of patients. Other duties include making telephone calls and answering them; as well as altering fire roll call registers. All in all, enrolled nurses seemed to carry out the more peripheral administrative duties, rarely being involved in the day-to-day decisions and running of the ward.

Administrative tasks for nursing auxiliaries again appear to be delegated tasks rather than individual responsibilities as part of the ward team. Clearly there was an emphasis placed on keeping nursing auxiliaries away from the office, unless they were carrying out specific delegated duties. These staff often bear the brunt of the patient workload; but are seen as having certain administrative skills "when it fits".

For example, nursing auxiliaries were frequently delegated such tasks as copying notes, drawn up usually by a registered nurse, from the patient's individual nursing notes into the daily report. Similarly, they would copy patients' shopping requests onto a central order sheet. Other clerical duties were of a similar delegated nature; and including fetching the staff duties list from the central office, and counting cutlery at meal times for purposes of security and safety.

Student nurses were not seen to interact in the administrative areas; which seems interesting, since nurse training should theoretically cover all aspects of ward routine and management.

Supervision of patients accounted for 25 per cent of time spent. The descriptive details follow. The clinical nurse specialist, together with the charge nurse, spent the least amount of time supervising patients. When they did this was often due to a shortage of staff; and consequently their involvement was from a security requirement rather than for therapeutic reasons.

Within this particular setting high levels of patient observation were required at certain times because of their potential dangerousness to themselves or others, especially since some were new to the hospital and had not received a full assessment. These peak times tended to be at rising; bathing; mealtimes; and preparing for bed. It was during these times that both charge nurse and clinical nurse specialists were involved in the supervision of patients. Main observations encountered consisted of observing patients rising and getting dressed; and observing patients shaving and showering. Both nursing grades also slipped back at times into the administrative role as required, and again once these peak observation times were complete.

The second predominant activity of staff nurses was that of supervising patients. Whilst also participating at peak times, similar to the charge nurse and clinical nurse specialist, there were considerable amounts of time that were spent in the general supervision of patients. These supervisory times reflected most parts of the day; and included mainly the supervision of patients whilst they were doing a variety of self-guided activities within their social time. These included watching television, playing games and other social pastimes.

It was difficult to decide during these observations how much, if any, of this social time of patients so avidly supervised was part of any therapeutic programme. Quite clearly there was therapeutic value in ensuring patients come to no harm to themselves or others. Quite often nurses were seen to be involved in dual activities. Thus staff were often observed watching television or reading newspapers or journals, whilst supposedly supervising or observing patients.

Clearly such dual activities, which essentially take concentration from the main task, are far from desirable. Again, once a particular task had been completed, such as supervising meals or doctors' visits, nurses seemed to revert back to supervision. Similarly, when supervision sessions ended, or to take a break from supervision, nurses returned to the ward office. It was evident that in most cases they did not return for instructions, but to reflect often on personal issues. Other supervisory interactions were observed; but these were relatively less frequent and consisted of opening sideroom doors and supervising medication rounds.

The observational activities both of enrolled nurses and nursing auxiliaries presented a similar picture. Both nursing grades interacted at peak times of patient movement, such as rising and bathing. However, it was quite clear that these nursing grades took the brunt of supervision of patients at other times consistently throughout the patients' waking day.

When "peak" times were over, the patients in most areas were left to do "their own thing" with appropriate supervision from nursing staff to ensure continuing safety. This leads to the suggestion that, outside of peak periods of patient movement or activity, there are long periods of time between approximately 0845 hours to 1200 hours, 1300 hours to 1630 hours and 1730 hours to 2145 hours, when patients are often left to their own devices without specific recreational or therapeutic involvement on the part of the nursing staff. This results in high proportions of staff "supervising" patients in a relatively non-interactive way.

The supervision of patients usually means that there is little if any interaction between staff and patient; resulting in little if any therapeutic input from the nursing staff. Little interaction is of a planned nature, either as nursing process activities or otherwise. As a result, nursing staff are usually just sitting or standing around during these periods; which in total account for some 25 per cent of the waking day. Again, dual activities were often observed, with staff frequently reading newspapers or watching television during supervisory activity.

Similarly, the supervision of patients also accounts for a proportion of student time. Whilst there are benefits in observing patient behaviours to acquire more experience and knowledge of health related conditions, the supervisory style adopted restricts more interactive therapeutic activity within the patient supervision category and has a clear impact on student nurse activity. If qualified nurses are to assist in student training then suitable role modelling is essential.

Nursing process activities

Nursing process interactions accounted for 16 per cent of ward observations. Charge nurses and clinical nurse specialists interacted most infrequently within this care area. Their dominance within the AS category was one of the main factors here; although, given more effective ward planning, there is no reason why their NP activities should not increase. Quite clearly the three staff involved at this level could better utilise their skills, and initiate improved patient care, if better resource management were implemented.

Staff nurses and enrolled nurses were far more involved in the nursing process than charge nurses and clinical nurse specialists. However, nursing auxiliaries were the staff who participated most in planned care for patients. Student nurses also interacted relatively infrequently within the nursing process category, their input being observational for learning in group situations rather than "hands-on" care involving student and patient. Details of the four phases of the nursing process and areas of interaction are discussed further, following Figure 10 (nursing process behaviours).

Patient social activities

Patient social activities in total accounted for 13 per cent of observed nurse behaviours. With regard to these, charge nurses and clinical nurse specialists participated least frequently; with the exception of student nurses, who were not observed socialising with patients. In the case of charge nurses, these behaviours mainly took place within two locations. The first of these was in the dayroom in the evenings, when both staff and patients often settled down to joint social activities such as board games and snooker. The second location was in the ward office, where interactions were initiated mainly by patients.

Observations of these grades socialising within the ward office supports the proposition that senior nursing grades are often reluctant to move away from their base to any degree. Observations within this area usually reflected patient-initiated conversation of a general nature (that is, discussing news or events; or passing the time of day). Social interactions within the dayroom for these grades tended to be rather different and of low frequency, and reflected a variety of social pastimes; although it is possible to speculate on whose benefit was paramount here. Examples of such activities are watching television programmes; and playing various games.

Staff nurses interacted considerably more with patients than either the charge nurse or the clinical nurse specialist. However, such interactions were limited to some degree by the "peripatetic" nature of the staff nurse's role. Unlike the charge nurse and nurse specialist, staff nurses were frequently out and about in other parts of the ward environment. Whilst social activities took place in a variety of locations within the ward, they mainly took place in two areas.

Most social interactions took place within the ward day room; and consisted mainly of watching television with patients, with some socialising discussion about the various television programmes. Other socialising events within this setting were games such as scrabble and cards, although these were less frequent. The other key social interaction tended to take place within the games room area. This activity was mainly playing snooker with patients and often contained social discussion throughout. Nurse-initiated interactions suggest that, to some degree, the precise nature of social activities may be biased towards staff interests and benefits, rather than those of the patients. Enrolled nurses and nursing auxiliaries interacted more frequently with patients than did other grades within the socialising areas. Both grades interacted with similar frequencies. Again, patient socialising activities took place mainly within the dayroom and games room areas of the ward. However, this is not to say that socialising with patients was not happening at other times and in other areas. As was the case with the staff nurses, similar interactive behaviours were observed; but it was evident that activities within this area were more varied for these staff groups. Activities within the dayroom included card games and related discussions; scrabble; and joking with patients. Games room activities were usually confined to snooker, which was the main activity in that area.

It became quite evident that certain staff have particular interests and related skills that are clearly beneficial to patients. However, it seems that these interests are only responded to by patients who have similar interests. Thus if a patient is to some degree motivated and has a specific interest, some form of interaction will be developed and hopefully some form of therapeutic benefit derived. This leaves a potential problem in that, if patients are not initially motivated, little if any interaction is offered.

Similarly, if the patient's health status restricts him from interacting, then he will receive little if any interactions. There appear to be great deficits here in terms of therapeutic intervention. In line with well-known social interactional and developmental theories, patients who are reasonably well and positively motivated will participate and benefit therapeutically from their interactions; whilst patients who are not so well are less interactive with staff (see, for example, Reed, 1978).

Reference was made earlier to the fact that no observations were recorded of student nurses socialising with patients. One variable may account for this. At the time of observation, student nurses were preparing for English National Board (ENB) assessments: and students may well have been using "socialising time" to prepare for these. The inference to be drawn here is quite clear. If student nurses are using time which should be devoted to clinical nursing experience to complete academic assessments, then important practical opportunities are being lost. It is essential that students gain related practical skills if they are to balance their theoretical knowledge.

Miscellaneous activities

Miscellaneous activities accounted for 9 per cent of ward observations. Whilst this category is unrelated to nursing care in any way, it should be looked at realistically when making ward improvements. This category is not a "catch-all"; and includes behaviours of a personal nature, such as making tea or visiting the toilet. These behaviours are an important part of daily life; and, provided they are not too frequent, can function to relieve tensions and stressors in a demanding environment.

Charge nurses showed the highest frequency of miscellaneous behaviours; with staff nurses, enrolled nurses, nursing auxiliaries and student nurses all showing similar frequencies. By far the most frequent activity was "visiting the toilet". Second was "reading newspapers" and "drinking tea"; and third were "general chit-chat" and "telephone conversation of a personal nature".

Because these behaviours are normative there seems little point in discussing them further. However, where staff are watching television and reading newspapers, this may be worthy of further comment. Such behaviours can rarely be acceptable within the context of patient supervision.

Patient functional activities

Patient functional activities accounted for some 7 per cent of total nursing activities. Charge nurses and clinical nurse specialists showed a lower frequency of such activities than other nursing grades in this area. Only at peak times would senior staff be involved in actually doing things for patients. "Peak times" are patients' rising; meal times; and bedtime, when there is a maximum number of patients moving around or concentrated in one area.

Activities tended to be in three areas. First and most frequent was serving meals to patients. This is an activity that could well be done by domestic staff; or possibly patients themselves could be more involved and benefit from the social learning situation which serving meals can provide. Second most frequent was giving medication, particularly during meal times. In many cases it appeared that meals were interrupted by this activity, which sometimes can be quite lengthy. There seems to be a tradition of giving medicines out during meal breaks; whereas some medications should or could be given prior to, or after, the meal.

Staff nurses displayed similar categories of activity: although their frequency and involvement was greater. Staff nurses' main PF activity was serving and giving meals. Similarly, medicines were given out by staff nurses during meal times. The only medicine round not to be given during meals was night-time medication. This latter practice was observed to be anti-therapeutic, due to the "regimental" queuing by patients which it engendered. Staff nurses' PF activities which did markedly differ from those shown by senior nursing staff were those concerned with actual "hands-on" care of patients. These included assisting with bathing and showering; as well as helping patients to shave and dress.

Enrolled nurses tended to be involved in most areas of PF activity. Generally activities were within the areas of assisting in serving meals and supervising medication: but rarely did enrolled nurses actually give out medication. Giving medicines was carried out mainly by staff nurses and occasionally by the charge nurse. Assisting with bathing and showering of patients was the most common feature of the role of the enrolled nurse in PF activities.

Nursing auxiliaries appeared mainly involved in one area of PF activity. These tasks all centred around the meal time. They included setting and laying tables; serving food; and clearing away dirty pots and assisting patients to complete their choice of menu. This was consistent throughout all meal breaks. It was interesting to note that nursing auxiliaries, who usually give the brunt of functional nursing care, were not observed to do more varied PF tasks for patients, such as helping them to wash or bathe.

Student nurses showed a similar pattern of involvement to that of nursing auxiliaries. Again they were frequently involved in serving and giving out meals; but were not observed to be involved in other PF aspects of care, as were staff nurses and enrolled nurses. However student nurses were involved with the dispensing of medicines.

Clinical education

Clinical education accounted for 5 per cent of activities for nursing staff. Clinical nurse specialists and student nurses interacted most frequently within this category. Student nurses' main activity within the learning situation was that of preparation for assessments and final examinations. These consisted of academic preparation for ENB Test B, particularly in consultation with the clinical nurse specialist.

Other frequent activities included reading the 1983 Mental Health Act; and dispensing medication under supervision of a first-line nurse. Other education-related activities consisted of attending medication lectures; and educational discussions with the clinical nurse specialist. It appeared that the clinical nurse specialist played a key role within nurse education, frequently in discussion with students and leading teaching sessions.

Charge nurses seemed to be rarely involved with students during the study periods; their only recorded CE behaviour was that of discussing student progress with the clinical nurse specialist. Other nursing grades interacted very infrequently with student nurses, this consisting in the main of supervision, particularly in relation to medication rounds; and students' approaching them for advice on a particular topic. Little formal education existed for nursing staff other than the student. This was usually self directed: such as reading one of the nursing journals. Despite the ward being a teaching ward, no visits or contact from education staff were recorded during the extensive observation period. This may particularly account for the lack of structured training or updating sessions for all ward nursing staff.

Domestic activities

Domestic behaviours were similar in frequency to those of clinical education; and accounted for 5 per cent of total behaviours. By far the most frequent behaviours within the domestic category were those of setting tables; making tea for patients; and clearing tables after meals. This tended to be done in the main by nursing auxiliaries, although very occasionally enrolled nurses assisted with table preparation. Staff nurses were involved relatively infrequently, usually clearing dishes away; collecting cutlery for security purposes; and assisting collecting dishes. Charge nurses tended to be involved in domestic inventories; and the clinical nurse specialist in ordering stock, although these behaviours were very infrequent. At no time during the observations were student nurses observed to carry out any domestic activities.

Once more there was an observed lack of patient involvement. Nurses were seen to be doing things that patients would find beneficial as part of their rehabilitation programme. Despite security and safety issues, it is simply not appropriate for patients to have *everything* done for them. The observation that only senior nursing staff were involved in ordering patient shopping may indicate some mismanagement of scarce nursing skills.

Nurse-patient behaviours

Quantitative analysis

Whilst there are many permutations of analysis that can be made using the customised database, Figure 8 (see next page) displays the analysis of individual behaviours. This subdivides the total observations in terms of (A) behaviours involving one-to-one nurse-patient interactions; (B) behaviours involving groups of staff and patients (group interactions); and (C) behaviours involving no direct nurse-patient interactions (indirect care). It is pointed out that, although category (C) behaviours show no evidence of interactions, care may well be at a planning stage when these occur.

As can be seen from figure 8, there are again broad similarities in nursing behaviours. Surprisingly in all wards (both internal and external) indirect care accounts for almost the same amount of time. These behaviours range from 63 per cent to 68 per cent, with a variance of plus or minus 2.5 per cent. These data suggest that on average nursing time is dominated by non-patient-involved activity for around 65 per cent of their time. Since an emphasis has been on a high ratio of qualified staff to each patient, these figures place much stress on the therapeutic value that such staff could offer when tied up with non-interactive duties.

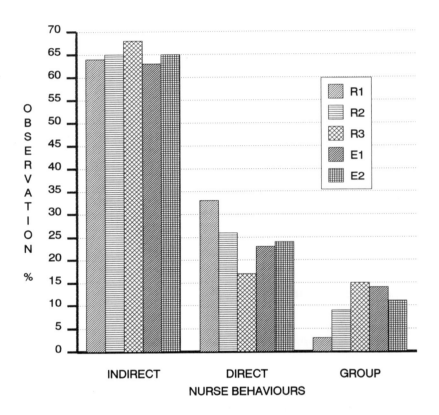

Figure 8 Nurse behaviour comparisons (internal and external locations)

Whilst some may argue that the observational instrument is insensitive to the changing activities of nursing staff, much of the data suggests otherwise. For example, when examining group and direct care, differing pictures emerge. Again, different types of ward reflect very different activities when it comes to individual patients. Direct care to patients ranges from 17 per cent to 33 per cent. In the case of R1 ward, one would expect the high frequency of one-to-one interactions observed; since this is a ward for female severely mentally impaired patients, and one would expect high levels of interactive input. Similarly, observed frequencies of group care are quite varied, ranging from 3 per cent to 15 per cent.

R1 ward accounts for the lowest frequency of group care. This is supported in practical terms, because people with severe learning disabilities often do not possess the skills to interact with one another, other than on a very short-term basis. In the case of R2 ward, one would perhaps not normally expect to observe high levels of one-to-one care on a ward that is essentially a pre-discharge environment. However, the high input of patient preparation in a variety of skills programmes, and especially games activities, immediately makes this understandable. Regarding group care, since individual patients are developing more personal autonomy ready for discharge, we can assume from the data that individuality is developing as personal confidence grows.

In the case of the external locations (E1 and E2 wards), both admission wards although within different health authorities, these data are supportive of previous observational frequencies; and do not show a variance for the various behavioural categories greater than plus or minus 1.5 per cent.

Psychiatric nursing activity seems to have embedded within it a whole range of supervisory and administrative tasks which take up over half of the nursing staff's time. When examining all areas of direct and group care, an interesting phenomenon emerges. Where a ward has a high frequency of direct care, it has a correspondingly lower frequency of group care. For example, in the case of R1, where direct care is high, there is a low level of group care. Similarly, where R3 has a medium frequency of direct care, it has a similar frequency of group care. These levels seem to rise and fall; yet the *indirect* care types remain fairly static.

It would now perhaps be useful to examine one of these wards in qualitative terms; and attempt to explain the different types of care within each of the care categories. First, as can be seen in Figure 9, indirect care accounts for 68 per cent of behaviours; with a sharp decline in frequency to 17 per cent direct care; and 15 per cent group care.

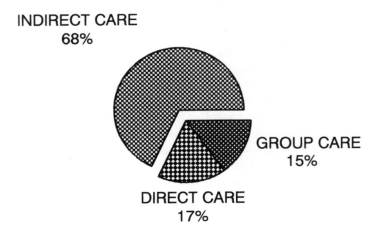

INDIRECT CARE
68%

GROUP CARE
15%

DIRECT CARE
17%

Figure 9 Nurse patient behaviours (Ward R3, N = 3000)

Qualitative interpretation

Indirect care

Indirect care to patients accounted for 68 per cent of behaviours for all nursing staff within the ward. However, it must be stressed that, although there is no contact between patient and nurse within this category, care could well be at a planning stage. Administrative activities and the supervision of patient behaviour accounted for most indirect care. Charge nurses and clinical nurse specialists were observed to spend the most time away from patient contact. Staff nurses spent less time within this category; although some of their behaviours were seen to be "intermediate" between indirect and direct modes of care.

Enrolled nurses and nursing auxiliaries figured very infrequently within the indirect care category; and only tended to be away from direct contact with patients when routine tasks occurred. Examples of indirect care involving charge nurses and clinical nurse specialists are administrative duties, such as answering telephones; dealing with ward staff and visitors; writing nurse's notes; and preparing case conference reports.

Indirect care for staff nurses appeared to be of two types: firstly, office-based duties, such as writing care plans and nursing notes and answering the telephone; and secondly, observing for security reasons disturbed patients who required careful observation, but did not necessarily need any interaction. Another frequently represented category was general observation of patients; and miscellaneous activities, such as reading newspapers and watching television.

Nursing auxiliaries and enrolled nurses tended not to be involved with administrative duties; and so were frequently in the presence of patients, but not necessarily interacting with them. Non-interactive behaviours involved supervision of patients and actually observing them for security and safety reasons. Student nurses tended to use these opportunities when little clinical interaction was occurring, usually between 0900 hours to 1200 hours and 1400 hours to 1630 hours, to concentrate on their training requirements such as ENB Test B work, which again impeded their contact with patients.

Group care

Group care to patients accounted for 15 per cent of nursing behaviours. Within this category patient socialising activities were the most frequent; with patient functional activities displaying similar frequencies. Other areas of group activity included supervision of patients; and domestic activities, which were relatively infrequent. Enrolled nurses and nursing auxiliaries most frequently interacted within group modes of care to patients. These consisted mainly, especially within the patient socialising areas of the ward, of playing cards or pool with patients. Other group activities were within the patient functional category, which often involved care of groups of patients at bathing and washing periods.

This last activity was especially relevant in the mornings, when nurses assisted several patients with washing or shaving. Unfortunately, task-orientated regimes contributed to patients being grouped together with little thought about individual programmes of care; privacy; dignity; or freedom of choice. Staff nurses, charge nurses and clinical nurse specialists did also interact in group care with patients; but these tended to occur in the evenings; and usually consisted of watching television with patients and playing games such as cards or scrabble. This again raises the issue of "whose benefit?". Student nurses only figured in one area of group care; that of patient functional activities, where they were involved in dispensing medications to groups of patients.

Direct care of patients on a one-to-one basis accounted for 17 per cent of observations. Direct care to patients was mainly within three behavioural categories: nursing process activities; patient socialising; and patient functional activities. It is of course recognised that it is not simply nursing process activities which may have a "one-to-one" nature. In terms of nursing process, theoretically patients could be involved in any of the four components, resulting in possible one-to-one interactions in assessment, planning, implementation or evaluation of care. In the current study, however, only implementation and assessments phases was found to result in one-to-one interactions involving patients and nurses.

Most interactions occurred in the implementation phase; with very few taking place during the assessment phase. Whilst all staff interacted with patients on a one-to-one basis some of the time, the nursing auxiliaries were clearly the staff who interacted the most frequently. Nurse-patient interactions involving nursing auxiliaries were frequently of a nursing process nature; especially those arising during the implementation phase. Other interaction consisted of patient socialising activities, such as playing games; and direct conversation with patients of a patient functional nature, whilst actually assisting him or her, for example in toileting or bathing.

Enrolled nurses similarly displayed NP-related behaviours; but not as frequently as the nursing auxiliaries. These were particularly involved with PF activities such as assisting secluded patients with their drinks; and with PS activities such as playing games with patients: e.g., snooker or cards. Staff nurses and charge nurses interacted with similar frequencies in most areas of one-to-one care with patients, such as NP and PS activities. It is interesting to note that nursing auxiliaries invariably drew the short straw when it came to PF activities such as bathing!

Charge nurses, clinical nurse specialists and staff nurses all displayed similar behaviours in relation to one-to-one care of patients. However enrolled nurses and nursing auxiliaries were rarely seen to include patients in assessments, especially in relation to the nursing process; and hardly ever undertook individual counselling work such as anger management; talking to newly admitted patients; or intervening with disturbed patients.

Current mental health policies place much emphasis on individual care for patients. The need for such guidelines becomes especially evident when, in the present study, observations show that, in both internal and external locations, time spent with patients accounts for only a maximum of 38 per cent of observed nursing activities; with only a modest proportion of this time accounting for nursing process activities.

With this finding in mind, we now examine the key features of nursing process activities within one ward setting.

Nursing process behaviours

Nursing process behaviours accounted for 16 per cent of total observations. Figure 10 (see next page) gives a breakdown of nursing behaviours and interactions to do with nursing process. Nursing process behaviours are categorised within the four phases, assessment; care planning; implementation; and evaluation. Each of these phases was further divided into "explicit" and "implicit" activities. "Explicit" behaviours are to do with verbal behaviours making explicit the activities occurring during any of the four phases; and "implicit" behaviours are any other behaviours (occurring at any stage of the process) from which NP activities may be implied, though not actually stated.

Figure 10 shows the frequency of behaviours within the eight nursing process codes: AE, AI, PE, PI, IE, II, EE and EI. The criteria for these codes can be found in Table 9 following. As can be seen assessment explicit (AE) behaviours account for 5 per cent of NP behaviours; and assessment implicit (AI) behaviours account for a further 8 per cent, giving a total of 13 per cent of behaviours relating to the assessment phase of the nursing process.

PLANNING EXPLICIT (PE) behaviours account for 1 per cent of NP behaviours and PLANNING IMPLICIT (PI) accounts for 0 per cent of NP behaviours; giving a total of 1 per cent of behaviours relating to the planning phase of the nursing process;

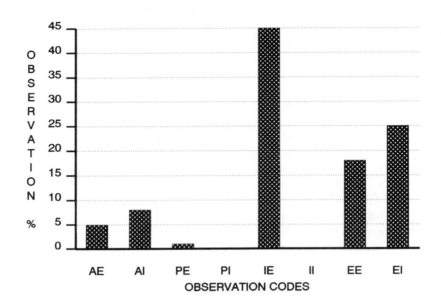

Figure 10   Nursing process behaviours (ward R3, 16% of total observations)

IMPLEMENTATION EXPLICIT (IE) behaviours account for 45 per cent of NP behaviours and IMPLEMENTATION IMPLICIT (II) behaviours account for 0 per cent of NP behaviours; giving a total of 45 per cent of behaviours relating to the implementation phase of the nursing process.

EVALUATION EXPLICIT (EE) behaviours accounted for 18 per cent of NP behaviours and EVALUATION IMPLICIT (EI) behaviours account for 25 per cent of NP behaviours; giving a total of 43 per cent of behaviours relating to the evaluation phase of the nursing process.

For an admission/assessment ward, there appeared to be little activity related to patient assessment. Whilst some discussion between nurses took place, only slightly more resultant activity actually occurred in regard to carrying out assessments. Similarly, the planning of care was almost non-existent. Qualitative analysis revealed that patients were often put onto a "maintenance" care plan that was predetermined for all patients. Whilst this may be a useful pragmatic strategy for introducing new patients to the ward, it denies the essentials of individual assessments and intervention.

The emphasis of nursing process activity was on implementation. Nurses were observed frequently in this category implementing a variety of self-help and personal hygiene care plans. What were clearly lacking in almost all cases were any care planning interventions based on direct care problems and on his/her reason for admission.

Table 9
Nursing process behaviour codes

AE (assessment explicit), that is, verbal behaviour to do with assessment of an individual patient.

AI (assessment implicit), that is, other behaviour by which assessment of an individual patient is IMPLIED, although not specifically mentioned;

PE (planning explicit), that is, verbal behaviour to do with care planning for an individual patient;

PI (planning implicit), that is, other behaviour by which care planning for an individual patient is IMPLIED, although not specifically mentioned;

IE (implementation explicit), that is, verbal behaviour to do with implementation of nursing care for an individual patient;

II (implementation implicit), that is, other behaviour by which implementation of nursing care for an individual patient is IMPLIED, although not specifically mentioned.

EE (evaluation explicit), that is, verbal behaviour to do with evaluation of nursing care for an individual patient;

EI (evaluation implicit), that is other behaviour by which evaluation of nursing care for an individual patient is IMPLIED, although not specifically mentioned.

It is essential that priority health-related problems are tackled first and directly related to the overall treatment plan. Evaluation of outcomes was high, when taking into account the low levels of assessment and planning. However, given that observed implementation and evaluation seemed to proceed with good effect, there seems to be no reason why the deficit areas cannot be rectified.

Observations of direct, one-to-one patient care were examined to determine whether they were patient-initiated or nurse-initiated. That is, is it patients that make demands or first move towards interaction? Or is it the nurse who initially interacts with the patient? Similarly, once the interaction starts, does the nurse reject it, tolerate it, or accept it completely? Table 10 shows the percentage of patient- or nurse-initiated interactions; and the pattern of rejection, toleration and acceptance related to these.

Table 10 Patient- and nurse-initiated interactions

INTERACTION TYPE:	R1:	R2:	R3:	E1:	E2:
PATIENT INITIATED INTERACTIONS	6%	36%	19%	11%	16%
NURSE INITIATED INTERACTIONS	94%	64%	81%	89%	84%

Table 10 demonstrates that interactions between patients and nursing staff are most frequently nurse-initiated. All wards, with the exception of R2 ward, show a similar nurse-initiated pattern. In the case of R1 ward, the nurse-initiated interactions are at a peak of 94 per cent. R2 ward shows a somewhat lower nurse-initiated ratio, attributable to the fact that this ward is a rehabilitation area, where it is expected that patients are becoming more independent in their preparation for discharge; resulting in a higher relative frequency of patient-initiated interactions.

Further qualitative analysis revealed that patients on R2 ward frequently interacted socially with nursing staff; and were clearly involved in long-established relationships with such staff. These relationships had been developed over a considerable period of time; and it is thought that the more relaxed environment of this pre-discharge ward plays a key role in developing these relationships. Similarly, it is hypothesised that, since the remaining wards are admission wards. By contrast, the high levels of nurse-initiated interactions occurring on R1 ward are readily seen as due to the perceived nursing needs of highly dependent, mentally impaired patients, who constantly require nursing intervention.

The findings illustrated in Table 10 show a clear domination of interactions by nursing staff. The remarkably low percentage of patients initiating interactions supports evidence presented elsewhere that patients are rarely actively involved with determining their care programmes. If patients' health status is to improve optimally, then it is essential that they become centrally involved in the processes of their own personal care. This, it is hypothesised, would lead to more balanced nurse-patient interactions. Figure 11 shows a more desirable, interactive care-initiated balance, which it is hoped would eventually "tip the scale" to a more optimal balance of nurse-initiated and patient-initiated interactions:

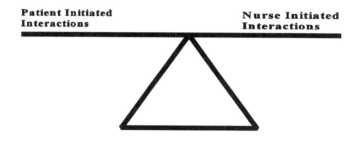

Figure 11 "Ideal" balance between patient and nurse interactions

Rejection, toleration and acceptance of interactions

Patterns of rejection, toleration and acceptance of interactions between nursing staff and patients were found to be essentially similar to those of nurse-initiated interactions. As can be seen in Table 11 overleaf, on only one ward (R1 ward) were any rejections of interactions observed. As indicated by the observer and reflected in the descriptive observational data, this was again attributable to the severe impairment of the patients, rather than to a problem associated with therapeutic input or nurse/patient relationships. All wards were observed to deliver substantially nurse-initiated therapeutic interactions that were in the main fully accepted by the patients. These accounted for between 91 and 98 per cent of interactions; with the exception again of R2 ward, where higher ratios of patient-initiated interactions were observed.

Table 11 Rejection, toleration and acceptance of
nurse-patient interactions

INTERACTION TYPE:	R1:	R2:	R3:	E1:	E2:
REJECTION OF INTERACTION	5%	0%	0%	0%	0%
TOLERATION OF INTERACTION	4%	22%	1%	3%	2%
ACCEPTANCE OF INTERACTION	91%	78%	99%	97%	98%

Whilst there was some toleration of interactions by patients in all five locations, those shown by patients in R2 ward accounted for a significantly higher proportion of 22 per cent. Qualitative analysis reveals some interesting phenomena which start to explain these behaviours. Almost all of the tolerations relate to over-confidence on the part of patients and their resultant inability to cope; at which point nurses may have to intervene.

Similarly, it is inferred that lack of support through appropriate care planning intervention is also a major contributor; in that patients may lack the skills to deal with socially significant issues. To give one example: a patient overspent his allocated money on a recent shopping excursion and found it difficult to cope when staff discussed issues with him following the event. Quite clearly the patient felt threatened by this situation and responded negatively to the interactions, consequently threatening the relationship. Had a care plan been developed prior to the shopping trip, with clear aims agreed by the patient, a more successful outcome would have resulted.

Use of language

Types of language used by nurses were analyzed to establish how they actually talked to patients, and in what style. Seven indicators were used to record the quality of language used by nurses to patients. These are given in Table 12 overleaf.

Table 12 Types of language used

1: INAUDIBLE TALK : the language is too quiet or the observer is too far away to hear it exactly.

2: ANGRY TALK: something said fiercely and angrily to the patient.

3: NEGATIVE CONTROL: don't do this or do that.

4: POSITIVE CONTROL: do this or that.

5: PROGRAMMATIC TALK: talking the patient through a specific course of action; explaining to him what he is doing whilst he is actually doing it.

6: EXPLANATORY TALK: language intended to make something clear to the patient.

7: EXPRESSIONS OF AFFECTION OR REGARD: gentle or considerate comments, or use of pet name.

The use of these types of language by nurses reveals some interesting data. The most frequent language types used by nurses in all five locations were expressions of affection and regard. Next most frequent, and almost similar in frequency, was the use of "explanatory talk". The use of this category was again consistent across all locations. Its main use related to nurses explaining aspects of social and work-related activities to patients.

For example, one patient was playing with a computer game; and did not understand a particular aspect relating to loading the programme. Following his request, a nurse then explained to the patient what he should do. Another patient was unsure how he should set out the dining room; and a nurse explained to him how he should carry this out. Explanatory talk was more frequent in R1 ward than any other linguistic category and explanation figured more frequently there then in any other location. Patients on this ward clearly required much input from nurses in explaining aspects of almost every daily activity.

As with care planning, the use of "programmatic talk" was relatively infrequent; and rarely occurred except on E1 ward. Whilst these examples could not be directly associated with care planning, there was clear use of language that involved the nurse talking a patient through a specific course of action. These programmes were wide and varied and included hair care; preparation of drinks; home visits; and moving rooms. Positive control was again infrequent in all locations with the exception of E1 ward, where staff were frequently heard to assist patients by the use of positive language prompts, such as asking the patient to remove his hat and coat; assisting the patient with the process of eating his lunch; and talking to a patient who was upset that he could not go home that weekend.

Negative and angry use of language was very infrequent. When it did occur, it appeared to be used in a more positive sense: for example, in asking a patient not to do something that was seen as developing into a possible danger to himself or to others. This use of language was heard more frequently on R1 ward than in any other location.

Most evident throughout observations was the infrequent use of any type of language with patients. Whilst we have looked briefly at what types of language nurses use with patients, it is equally important to mention that most frequently no conversations took place with patients. One good example of this for all five locations is that of patient supervision. This activity, which accounted for approximately 20 per cent of nurses' time, was seldom accompanied by any attempt to converse with the patients. When it did occur, it was usually patient-initiated.

Some observations indicated that certain patients would request some nursing intervention; but were frequently ignored by the nurse until their behaviour escalated to an "unacceptable" level. The use of appropriate language, possibly prescribed in relevant care plans, could play a significant role here that would assist in preventing these long periods of potentially stressful silence. In addition, nurses seemed not to know what to say or do within these situations. As with relatively poor levels of care planning skills, resulting in low levels of care planning activity, education is clearly lacking in the use of language as a "therapeutic agent" with which to improve the quality of patient care.

Non-verbal indicators

Non-verbal indicators were examined for positive and negative use of body posture. No negative gestures were found in any of the five locations. Only positive use of body movements was found within the locations; although these too were relatively infrequent. Nurses appeared rarely to use their body movement to support any verbal explanations. Occasionally, use of hand and arm movements was observed; but these were mainly used as additional support to verbal responses, such as programmatic or explanatory talk.

Emic and etic issues

Similarities in quantitative terms have been discussed in relation to Figures 6 and 8. These figures offer an emergent general picture of psychiatric nursing. These similarities are consistent within both internal and external contexts. However, quantitative comparisons only serve to inform in broad terms; but cannot give details about the exact qualitative nature of such similarities and differences. Qualitative analysis of the eight care categories reveals a generic similarity between "mainstream" psychiatric nursing care and the forensic psychiatric nursing care encountered within Rampton Hospital.

Administrative activities:

Administration both internally and externally differed very little. Most administrative duties, such as dealing with doctors; filling in nursing notes; and dealing with telephone calls were consistent throughout all the wards. Only one psychiatric ward differed to any degree. On E1 ward, AS behaviours were observed less frequently due to the more advanced multidisciplinary approach in use there, resulting in other disciplines carrying out their share of care recording.

Similarly, this ward showed a high level of co-ordinated multidisciplinary care that did not always require the presence of nursing staff. Psychiatric nursing appears to have less effect on patients because highly skilled and trained staff are tied up carrying out AS duties. Whilst some of these duties may be necessary, much could be delegated to differently qualified members of staff; or would be more appropriate to an administrative assistant.

The redirection of resources is a vital component of ward management with which ward managers and charge nurses should become more familiar. The tying-up of often scarce nursing resources in the performance of inappropriate tasks can only limit the continuing health care process for patients; and serve as a frustrator for nursing staff who lack opportunities to apply highly developed professional skills.

Patient supervisory activities

Whilst the supervisory aspects of patient care differ within the Rampton Hospital contexts because of the potential dangerousness of patients, patient supervisory activities tended to be quite similar in all locations. Generally, there seemed to be a situation in which nurses sat around for considerable lengths of time, "observing" patients, but rarely interacting with them. These data suggest that nurses are frequently unsure what to do with patients, often waiting for patients to do something, so they can respond. Patients often make repeated attempts at attention-seeking before nurses intervene.

The whole philosophy of this type of nursing care seems to be underpinned by the nurse's need to leave the patient to his own devices. The only supervisory aspect of patient care that differs to any degree is the high level of security which is present within Rampton Hospital. Worthy of comment here is the frequent observation of care practices which cater for role abridgement, rather than operating on the basis of individual patient needs.

Patient functional activities

Patient functional activities, whilst obviously differing in relation to the physical and psychological demands of patients, were also generically similar. The common theme here was that nurses in all locations tended to "overcare" for patients. This was particularly evident on R1 ward, where the patients were suffering from severe learning disabilities. Whilst still evident in external wards, it was not quite as frequent there as in the Rampton context.

"Overcaring" for patients involves doing things for patients rather than encouraging them to "do it for themselves". The data suggest that psychiatric nursing is still largely based on a task-oriented approach that has not focused adequately on the patient as an individual, despite the introduction of care planning.

Patient social activities

These activities were similar in frequency across all locations, as was the case with other behavioural categories. The only significant difference apart from frequency was that of the type of social activity. Personal social activity, such as chit-chat and the use of greeting phrases such as "Good morning", were more frequently encountered on E1 ward. The other external ward (E2) showed very infrequent social verbal communications with patients.

In general, the internal locations showed similar patterns of PS behaviour to those encountered in the external locations. The only other difference was in the type of social activities undertaken. These consisted largely of simple variations in a repertoire of card or board games, rather than any major difference in approach. Also worthy of note is that, as patients become more independent, socialising activities appear to increase, as was the case on R2 ward. Clearly, the more relaxed atmosphere and pre-discharge ambience are key variables here.

Domestic activities

Domestic behaviours did not vary to any great degree, apart from on R3 ward, where nurses tended to do things for patients in a domestic capacity, rather than encourage patients to do things such as clearing away dinner pots for themselves. Similar features were observed in all the Rampton Hospital wards, where the observer would frequently see nurses doing things for patients who, given the opportunity and appropriate support, might well have done things for themselves. In addition, the Rampton nurses frequently carried out routine domestic chores such as cleaning and clearing away.

By contrast, in the external locations, patients were encouraged more to do things for themselves. Similarly, despite their mental health problems, patients appeared more capable of carrying out such daily chores. In all locations nurses spent a considerable time in domestic duties, such as cleaning; preparing food and drinks; and clearing away dirty pots when domestic help was available. Valuable nursing skills are again lost here; and more effective use of these is required.

Miscellaneous activities

This category was significantly higher within the external locations although frequencies differed. Whilst there were similarities within this category, such as reading newspapers, making tea, and personal issues such as using the toilet, there was one major difference. E2 ward had a culture which meant that, at peak times such as patient rising - when the demand on nursing skills would be at its highest - nursing staff were often seen to be taking coffee and breakfast breaks.

These were carried out in isolation from patients. However, patients were occasionally observed going to the staff room and communicating with nurses. Quite often nurses were seen to take these breaks for periods of up to one hour; with rarely more than one nurse left in real contact with patients. Regarding the internal locations, behaviours were broadly similar to those seen in the external locations; but staff were not seen to be leaving patients unsupervised. Possibly the stricter supervision of security and safety issues within the Rampton Hospital context plays an important role here.

Clinical education

Whilst quantitative data show broad similarities, this behavioural category reveals some interesting differences. Education in the external ward locations was largely dependent on team-orientated student learning. Students were involved (particularly on E1 ward) in various tests relating to their training. In addition most clinical education was self-directed, with some practical support from ward-based nurses.

In the Rampton Hospital locations, apart from R1 ward, clinical education appeared to depend almost exclusively on the nurses reading various journals and books; although one location (R3 ward) saw some input from the clinical nurse specialist. As with the external locations, R1 ward staff were very much involved with, and supportive to, student members of the ward team. What was not observed in any location were any planned education programmes for nursing staff other than students. Similarly, no observations were made of tutorial visits by education staff.

Nursing process activities

These behaviours were greater in frequency within the internal contexts than in the external. It is thought that the nursing process coordinators had been a significant influencing variable here. External locations were both similar regarding relative frequencies; with implementation occurring more frequently than the other phases. Similarly, the internal locations showed implementation of care accounting for the highest frequency of nursing process behaviours.

Qualitative analysis revealed a marked difference in the types of patient care planning programmes. The internal care programmes dealt mainly with personal problems in daily living, such as bathing, personal hygiene and social programmes. In most cases, when compared with the reason for admission, these did not relate to the patient's priority health problem(s). By contrast, external care plans tended to be directly related to the patient's reason for admission; and were based on a formal assessment and prioritisation of needs.

Relationship of care planned to that actually given

All locations were examined to assess if the care that was planned within the nursing process documentation was actually given. Planned interventions were compared with progress notes reflecting what nurses said they had done; and these were both compared with observations of care actually given. Within all locations there was no doubt that care recorded was actually given, although some anomalies were observed. Both in internal and external locations there was what appeared to be an "unplanned" approach to implementing planned care.

Despite "key nurse" responsibilities, there seemed little if any coordination concerning when to deliver planned care. Within each location patients often displayed behaviours that demanded care plan intervention; but only received input after several demands, or when the behaviour became intolerable to the nursing staff. The documented progress notes on planned care revealed both the greatest similarities and the greatest deficits. All documentation reflected a variety of skills. Only that produced by R2 ward appeared to be more concise and informative. This was thought to be due to recent educational input on care planning on that ward.

All sets of progress notes again reflected varied levels of skills. Whilst some recordings were clear and concise and reflected care intervention that was empirically observed, others were of a nature that could not be related to care planning. These were recordings of interventions that could not be compared with planned care. Typical were entries which read : "... Tommy had a good day today". These are global statements which do not represent the care given; or, perhaps even more importantly, any specific patient response or outcome.

5 Innovation in observational data collection and analysis

Overview

This section describes some advances in electronic data capture and analysis developed in connection with observational aspects of the study. It updates observational methodological advances and findings from studies carried out in 1993, providing useful comparisons with the main body of data collected in 1990.

Hand-held computers in clinical audit (Robinson, 1993)

The paper-and-pencil method of recording observational audit data during this study (Robinson, 1988) was found to be extremely time consuming, especially in manual analysis; re-inputting data to database for analysis; and producing the final report. In fact, it is becoming increasingly common for audit results to take several weeks, if not months, to feed back. Similarly, research reports can take years to complete and are sometimes out of date when completed.

In particular, this study collected 15,000 observations. Every 400 observations took approximately six hours to re-input to the database. This equals a total of more than 225 hours spent re-inputting data. Influenced by the study of Reed and Dean (1990), the researcher gave considerable thought to the possible application of hand-held computers for capturing data at the source. If this were possible, potentially all these hours could be saved.

Following lengthy reviews and trials with hand-held computers and the successful capture and transfer of pilot data, the researcher hypothesised that the use of hand-held computers and related database would significantly reduce the time for data analysis and report feedback.

Little research has so far been undertaken on the use of hand-held computers for this type of data capture; though potential benefits are considerable, given an effectively conceptualised database and due attention to related education and change strategies (Reed and Dean, 1990). The literature reveals that although some work has been carried out using hand-held computers (for example, Flowers, 1982; Lechl et al, 1988; Lewis et al, 1985; Sanbury et al, 1985) little is health care related. Where it is, recording tends to be quantitative (Greenhalgh, 1992); with few if any capturing a descriptive style of input (Reed and Dean, 1990; Flowers, 1982); or applying this within the clinical audit setting or research data collection.

Following further trials and literature reviews, a proposal was put forward and subsequently accepted for funding within the Department of Health audit allocation monies. The £44,000 funded both equipment and a nurse researcher for two years. This two-year research project (Curl, Robinson and Reed, 1992) carried out an in-depth comparison of paper-and-pencil and hand-held data recording methods; and assesses the implications for their use in both clinical practice and support services. The main aims of the programme were to:

Develop hand-held computers for use in capture and upload of observational data;

Compare efficiency of hand-held computers with traditional pencil-and-paper methods;

Assess implications of the study for use in wider multidisciplinary and support service contexts.

Subsequently a programme was developed which had three distinct components that integrate into an observational audit package which has the capabilities of next-day feedback of results and, it is predicted, will exert a significant influence on future data collection methods.

Customised database

A data collection and storage facility was developed using Masterfile PC database. The computer software is a commercially available database. The application of this software allows collection of information about how patients are cared for, correlating this information, and analysing it in various ways. Most of these applications are automatic, so only a minimal knowledge of how to use a computer is necessary.

The program was designed around the Ward Observation Schedule used in the present study, with the data collection fields customised into the programme. Analysis of data also required to be considered during this development to design the programme efficiently. Fifteen data fields were programmed into the database, based upon the data to be collected. This programme would then serve two purposes: first, as the electronic programme for the hand-held computer in which to collect the data; second, the subsequent receiving database for analysis. The data collection fields are given in Table 13.

Table 13 Data collection fields in customised database

Date
Time
Staff Grade
Staff Code
Patient Code
Description of Activity
Activity Code
Indirect/group/direct care type
Rejection/toleration of interaction
Patient/nurse initiated interaction
Language type used by nurse
Non-verbal indicators
Location of activity
Number of staff present in area
Number of patients present in area

The database for analysing these data is designed to allow fast, reliable data comparisons within clinically important parameters set out in Table 13. From these data, it is possible to calculate and compare any of the data fields collected; for example, a particular activity on any day of the week or time of day by staff grade; staff/patient ratios; skill mix or patient interactions at specific times or on specific days. Any number of the identified fields can be compared with each other. In addition, key words or phrases for qualitative detail can also be searched for and compared by means of string-scanning techniques (see Annexe J).

For purposes of making these comparisons, the types of data analysis required were examined; and twenty-four initial comparisons were identified, although these can be further expanded. Consequently, the database was programmed to calculate these twenty-four comparisons; and the whole routine assigned to just one key press. Calculations take only a few minutes and the database can be revisited at any time for additional information or qualitative detail. To access information the data can either be displayed on the screen or printed out using a report generator.

Report generator

The report generator is an extension of Masterfile PC database, in which calculated data can be assigned to predetermined template reports. Templates showing relevant details were programmed for each of the twenty-four sets of analysis. These templates form the report to which the calculated data is assigned. For example, Template 3 will access the database for the pre-calculated data and assign it to the report as a frequency; a percentage; and, if required, as a ratio. This is then either dumped to the VDU screen or printed out as hard copy. An example of a template report with assigned frequency and percentage is given in Figure 12, following :

RAMPTON HOSPITAL QUALITY ASSURANCE DEPARTMENT Report 3: TOTAL WARD OBSERVATIONS		
Description of Care Observed:	Frequency:	Percent:
Communication WITH patient	459	17.67
Communication ABOUT patient	99	3.81
Direct CP activity	407	15.67
Indirect CP activity	69	2.66
Patient-functional	2	0.08
Patient-social	60	2.31
Routine medications	87	3.35
Group therapy	6	0.23
Patient supervision ON WARD	416	16.01
Patient supervision OFF WARD	38	1.46
Administration ON WARD	664	25.56
Administration OFF WARD	47	1.81
Clinical Education	38	1.46
Domestic	74	2.85
Personal	132	5.08
TOTALS:	2598	100.00

Figure 12 Template report with assigned frequencies and percentages

The care constructs above are slightly different from those presented in the observational findings section.   This was a result of the natural construct progression resulting in new empirical care categories being identified and subsequently modified. This natural progression is highlighted in the final section of this report.

Hand-held computer trials

Following detailed review of currently available hand-held terminals, the DIP 512k pocket PC was used in preliminary trials to establish the working logistics of the programme. The associated database (Masterfile PC) was adapted sufficiently to run on this machine. Trial data were successfully input and downloaded, with a minimum time-saving of one minute for each four observations. Since approximately 600 observations were required to secure a realistic ward profile, this represented a minimum time-saving of approximately six to eight observer hours for each clinical ward audit.

The database was customised to run on the forty-column screen of the hand-held computer. The purchase of a new full-screen version of the hand-held computer (Sharp 3100) eliminated earlier screen restrictions encountered with the DIP 512k.

The programme for inputting data into the hand-held computer was designed to be extremely user-friendly and this computer consequently operable by people with a minimum amount of computer skills. For example, each field (see Table 13) is displayed in turn by the computer and is designed to prompt the operator for the required data. Once this is input, the operator is prompted for the next; and so on, until data collection is complete. An example of one of the data fields as seen on the computer screen is shown in Figure 13.

ENTER DESCRIPTION OF ACTIVITY
Nurse showing patient how to dress herself whilst explaining what to do

---

Figure 13 The computer screen prompts for each answer

Comparing electronic data capture with paper and pencil technique

Data were collected on three wards, using both paper-and-pencil and hand-held computer techniques for recording. Each method consisted of four weeks data collection per ward, with a total of approximately 2,400 observations collected using each technique in each location. Each observation consisted of up to fifteen data field entries. Detailed note taking of times taken for each phase, as well as the practicalities, benefits and problems, was carried out following each observation period. Data loss between the two methods has been negligible in that it is possible to collect a similar amount by both methods. Obviously, the practicalities of this are in the time-saving of not having to re-input data into the main database.

Uploading electronic data

Data transfer to the main computer and database takes place by copying data to the A drive storage card of the hand-held computer. This is then uploaded into the main computer using a card drive attached to it. The whole routine takes just seconds. Calculations of the data were programmed into the database; and the whole operation assigned to one key. Thus once data are collected and uploaded to the main computer, assuming there is no input error, calculations can be done in minutes. For example, the 2,400 observations, each containing fifteen data fields or entries, are calculated against twenty-four predetermined sets of analysis. This is done at the rate of 1,000 per minute or less. Once calculations are complete, they are simply assigned to the report generator for printing out (see Figure 12).

Automatic error checking

In the initial stages of data analysis and subsequent computer report, printing errors had a dramatic effect on the printing of reports. Unrecognised inputs would confuse the automatic analysis and slight miscalculations would occur. Errors, however, represented only a minor proportion (approximately 30 out of 36,000 inputs, or less than 0.2 per cent). However careful human operators are at trying to enter information accurately, they will always make some mistakes! In order to minimise the effects of wrong data giving erroneous results when they are analyzed, several automatic error-traps have been incorporated into the application. The mistakes, or omissions, will not necessarily be corrected by the computer; but at least there are now some easy ways to find the errors and put them right.

These have been designed to show information when the data has been left out, or wrongly recorded. The screen automatically shows an error message if data are outside the parameters which it is programmed to accept. For example, if a code D1 to D2 is required to be input, and an input of E1 is entered, an error will be shown. Errors cannot be detected if D1 is entered instead of D2. Errors may also be seen on the Data Input Screen. Once these are detected they can be highlighted and rectified.

Patient benefits

The observational measure used within the project is able to measure care practices in a way that has so far been relatively unexplored. It provides precise details of nurse and patient interactions that are not only measured quantitatively; but also the qualitative detail of what actually happened can now be teased out. These fine details of patient care will contribute to the constant quality improvement of clinical care to patients; and allow suitable change and education strategies to be implemented. The rapid feedback of data means that the data are much more relevant and clinically "real", since next-day feedback can be achieved. Similarly, final report data are much more relevant and appropriate to the time they were collected; ensuring that change strategies are based upon current data.

General benefits

Hand-held electronic data capture is proving to be acceptable, reliable and qualitatively as rich as paper-and-pencil methods. The developing observational audit package (Computerised observational care audit) using these computers complements user-friendly software that allows rapid analysis and report feedback following data collection. The use of hand-held computers will represent a critical advance in multidisciplinary data collection and upload. In addition, spin-offs for other types of data collection in a variety of settings will be of great potential benefit. Benefits emerging include:

Rapid feedback of results;

Considerable savings on observer time inputting data manually to main database;

Reduction of opportunity for data input errors;

Error-free data transfer to main database, improving reliability of collected data;

Fast, efficient transfer of data to main database;

Increase in confidentiality and security of data transfer by elimination of paper-and-pencil stage;

Potential for multidisciplinary data collection;

Capture of qualitatively rich data, providing precise details of clinical care and related activities;

Potential use in all areas of audit data collection.

Clearly there is great potential for hand-held computers in collecting audit data at source. Within this programme using observational measures, time-savings of up to three days were established during each of the data collection periods. Similarly, with the electronic database and report generator, additional substantial time-savings were gained. Most importantly, the collection of data electronically at source, the instant transfer of data, rapid analysis and report generating all contribute to results being fed back to the clinical area within a day of final data collection.

Currently, we have now gained much information about the application of hand-held computers in the clinical setting, although it will be a while before the final report is complete. However, current feelings are extremely positive regarding the method's high potential within all areas of care audit.

Not all has been plain sailing since battery life; customisations to software; programming; and "getting-to-grips" with new technology presented numerous problems. These difficulties have been largely overcome through continuous evaluation and modifications. Recently hand-held computers have been introduced within medical audit at Rampton Hospital; and catering audit is to be developed shortly. Currently, a collaborative venture with general nursing is under way following validation of care constructs for the general nursing context (see section nine for results and comparisons).

Baseline measures for female personality disorder unit

As a result of the hand-held computer programme a package was developed which could be used both within Rampton Hospital and in wider contexts. This package (Computerised Observational Care Audit) was used within the female personality disorder unit (PDU) programme to examine the care context prior to the development of the ward. The ward (R4) is a twenty-bedded female ward with patients suffering from a wide variety of personality disorders. Nursing staff include both men and women.

Following two weeks of careful groundwork and familiarisation with the ward team, patient and routine data were collected over a four-week period. Quantitative data analysis using twenty predetermined reports was carried out upon completion of data collection; and next-day feedback of results achieved. Qualitative details of the data were analysed and fed back to the ward one week later.

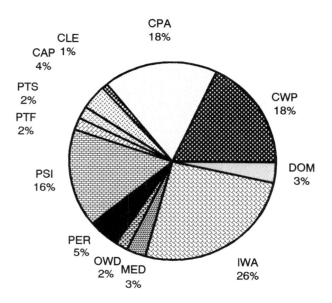

Figure 14 Total ward observations (Ward R4, N = 2598)

Quantitative analysis

As can be seen in Figure 14, (above) a similar picture to that presented in the previous main study observational findings is present, despite some differences in the changing care constructs. The key to the figure differs slightly from that presented earlier and the revised version can be found following the figure (see Table 14). In-ward administration activities (IWA) accounted for 26 per cent of nursing activity, with communication with the patient (CWP) and care plan activity accounting for 18 per cent. Patient supervision (PSI) accounted for 16 per cent of activities; with a further decrease to personal activities (PER) at 5 per cent.

We now see a levelling-out of behaviours to communicating about the patient (CAP) accounting for 4 per cent of nursing activity. Medication (MED) and domestic activities (DOM) both occur with a similar frequency of 3 per cent; and patient social (PTS), patient functional (PTF) and off-ward duties each account for 2 per cent. Of the remaining two behavioural categories, clinical education (CLE) accounts for 1 per cent and group therapy (GPT) for 0.2 per cent (NB: this last is not shown within the figure because it is too small to interpret).

103

Table 14 Revised behavioural codes

CWP (communication with patient): Any one-to-one communication with a patient, by word or sign, about any topic, other than care plan activity. Examples include, casual conversation, talking a patient through an activity, giving directions to a patient and collecting information from the patient.

CPA (care plan activity): Any verbal or non-verbal behaviour relating to the individual care plan. Examples include, assisting the patient to carry out an assessment or making an assessment, planning care, implementing the plan, evaluation and completing progress notes.

PTF (patient-functional): Any general, task-orientated, physical care of patients, unrelated to an individual care plan (actually doing things for or assisting patients).

PTS (patient-social): Behaviours relating to task-orientated social care of patients, unrelated to an individual care plan. Examples include, playing games, watching TV or general chit-chat with patients.

GPT (group therapy): Taking part in, running or acting as co-worker, in a therapy group. These are groups with a direct therapeutic purpose, rather than simply general social groups. Examples include, counselling or anger management groups.

MED (medication): Administering medication, either as part of a medicine round, depot injection or on a PRN basis. Other examples include, reading medicine cards or filling them in.

PSI (patient supervision on the ward): Staff supervision of patients within the ward, but not participating in care plan activity: eg, sitting in the dayroom with patients, moving patients from room to room within the ward, or unlocking a door, seeing a patient through it and locking it again.

CAP (communication about patient): Any verbal behaviour relating to a patient but not actually involving the patient or concerning his/her care plan. Examples include, staff discussions about patient in general terms, or related to his/her health status, with any member of the clinical team.

IWA (in the ward administration): Any discussion, paperwork or other behaviour that contributes to the running of the ward, but not to any individual care plan: eg, filling out menus, meeting visitors, answering general telephone calls, filling in documents or filing them, giving instructions to staff.

(Table 14 continued)

DOM (domestic): Behaviours and discussions related to ward domestic arrangements rather than to patients. These may be related to, or involve carrying out ward cleaning or storage of items such as laundry, and serving food.

PER (personal): Any verbal or non-verbal behaviours of a personal nature: eg, eating, drinking, going to the toilet, reading the newspaper or general chit-chat unrelated to the ward.

CLE (clinical education): Any discussions or behaviour relating to any aspect of nurse education, involving any member(s) of the nursing team, including students). Examples may include, participating in seminars, ward discussions, nurse- or tutor-led sessions, undertaking tests or other learning experiences.

OWD (off-ward duties): Any behaviour relating to ward management taking place outside the ward. Examples include, collecting drugs from pharmacy, collection of files, taking patients to X-ray or other services.

LOB (level of observation): Any verbal or non-verbal behaviour that relates to the observation, documentation and communication of patients who require close observation. These should include observations that are care-plan related. Examples include level 2 and 3 observations; seclusion; completing related documents; and discussion of such a patient's health status.

Nursing behaviours

Figure 15 shows nursing behavioural interactions in terms of: direct care, consisting of one-to-one interactions between nurse and patient; group care, involving groups of staff and patients; and indirect care, indicating no interaction between staff and patients. However, although no interaction may take place in the indirect care type, care could still be at a planning stage.

The theme continues within Figure 15, in that we have seen these patterns of care emerging in previous chapters. Contact with patients through direct and group types of care shown here is a pattern identified earlier and accounts for 60 per cent of total nursing behaviours. These patterns indicate that nursing delivery and time is still largely uncoordinated and unplanned. Similarly these data, which are essentially up to date, show little difference from those collected in the pilot and main studies, which together go back some six years (ROBINSON, 1987, 1989).

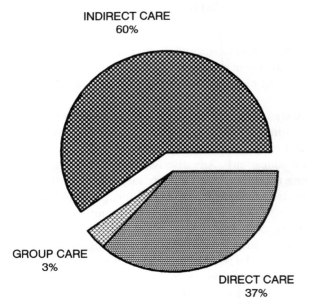

INDIRECT CARE
60%

GROUP CARE
3%

DIRECT CARE
37%

Figure 15 Nurse patient behaviours (Ward R4)

Qualitative analysis: Data unrevealed through quantitative description

Whilst not wishing to go over ground previously covered, a qualitative look at key areas will follow, to give examples of descriptive care processes.

Care planning activity

Direct care planning activity relates to 18 percent of observations. Level 3 observations relate to disturbed patients who require individual direct observation and barriers should not interfere due to the nature of the patient under constant observation. Whilst it is clear that there is considerable assessment and evaluation taking place, these particular data reflect a lack of planning, but more significantly a lack of any therapeutic intervention.

Approximately 2 per cent of the 18 per cent was related to direct care interventions such as counselling. The remaining 16 per cent related to direct observations of Level 3 patients. It is worth noting that frequently within Level 3 observations nurses were engaged in dual activity. The important factor here is that, whilst Level 3 observations were recorded in care plans, very little actual intervention occurred. At a time when patients clearly required careful input and support, very little was given. In other words, Level 3 observations written into care plans frequently led to nothing more than a therapeutically inactive nursing presence.

It is also worth noting at this stage that the documentary analysis was used just after this period of data collection to assess the status of care planning within the ward. The results showed that care planning was at a very primitive stage and needed major input from educationalists.

Communication with patient

This category accounted for 18 per cent of ward observations. However, it was noted that of these 65 per cent were patient-initiated interactions. These included requests by patients, such as bedroom door locking/unlocking, asking for cigarettes or informing staff about something. Few were related to care planning.

Group therapy

This category accounted for only 0.2 per cent of nursing activities. It was interesting to note that though supposedly the "type" of patient within R4 Ward "tends not to mix in groups", the data suggest that the four patients within this category were part of a handicraft group that appeared to progress positively. The inference is that this type of group work might well be developed with future advantage to patients.

Domestic

This category accounted for 3 per cent of ward observations. Qualitative details reveal tasks such as clearing away and washing pots; making drinks; emptying bins; clearing away tables; tidying the kitchen; attending to laundry; an interesting phenomenon, since there appears to be considerable domestic help also available on this ward.

Clinical education

This category accounted for 1 per cent of ward observations. This category was mainly student oriented and consisted of nurses, and at one point a psychologist, assisting with a programme of student training. Other attributes related to student self-directed activities. Topics encountered within this category were care planning; aspects of Project 2000; distribution of medication; and legal aspects of care. Whilst tutorial contact was made with the student, no input was seen in terms of clinical education for the remaining ward team during the observed period, despite the fact that this ward had an identified development programme.

In-ward administration

This category was by far the most dominant activity, accounting for over one-quarter of staff time (that is, 26 per cent of ward observations). Whilst this category includes the general administration and running of the ward, there were some interesting areas of involvement which, if freed up, would allow more nursing time to be spent in patient care. These activities included dealing with both internal and external incoming and outgoing telephone calls; filling-in menus; constructing posters/notices; tidying the ward office; dealing with income/outgoing mail; ordering clothes and food; and by far the most frequent involved nursing staff dealing with ward visitors, which accounted for 15% of in-ward administrative activity.

Patient supervision

This category accounted for 16 per cent of ward observations. Qualitative analysis revealed nurses making general observations of patient care; but during the majority of observations there was a complete social distance between patients and staff; with nurses frequently grouped together away from patients. This period of general observation of patients was also used to carry out a variety of other activities, such as writing reports; reading newspapers; chatting to other staff; and responding to patients' requests. The main period where nursing staff tended not to carry out dual activity was during the period of patient meal breaks.

Off-ward administration

This category accounted for 2 per cent of ward observations. This category relates to general administration regarding the running of the ward; and often consisted of going on errands. These involved nursing staff making trips to areas such as the sewing room; returning security radios; photocopying; collecting the pet fish (!); meetings on other wards; and nursing development meetings. Frequently these activities tied up qualified staff rather than nursing auxiliaries.

Time period analysis

Communication with patients (CWP) appears to occur least frequently during the early morning period of commencing observations at 0730-0759 hours; between 0800-0859 hours; and between 1400-1459 hours. Care planning direct (CPD) appears fairly constant throughout most of the day, apart from significant increases during the period 1300-1359 hours, 1400-1459 hours, 1500-1559 hours and 1600-1659 hours. Since this particular care planning activity relates mainly to Level 3 observations, further investigation is needed to determine why Level 3 observations almost double their frequency within these time periods. Perhaps this may give some insight into the appropriate interventions and preventive behaviours needed to reduce the necessary frequencies of this activity.

The patient supervisory category (PSI) reveals that there was minimal staff presence with patients during the first two time periods. This significantly increases from 0900 hours onwards; but a marked difference exists during the periods 1100-1159 hours and 1300-1359 hours. For some reason during these two periods there is constant presence with patients. Qualitative analysis of these two categories reveals nurses being present in a supervisory rather than an interactive capacity. Dual activities, for example, staff/patient discussions, reading newspapers and watching television were frequently encountered.

During the "low" period of patient supervision within the first two time bands, there is quite clearly a significantly higher percentage of ward administration activity (IWA). It appears that nursing staff are then concentrating perhaps more on administrative duties than on supervising patient care. Ward administration for these two time bands is as high as twice the total ward average. Similarly there appear to be high levels of ward administrative activities within the last time band of the waking day.

6 Findings of the documentary analysis

Documentary analytic checklist: quantitative application

Each nursing care plan from the three internal and two external locations (N=50) was subject to detailed analysis using the specially-designed, fifty-six-item checklist (Robinson, 1988; see Annexe B). This instrument incorporates each stage of the nursing process (assessment; care planning; implementation of care and evaluation) in four discrete sections. Each of the fifty-six checklist items was applied in turn to the care plan and related documents. Based on the scoring criteria, it is possible to derive a cumulative score relating to each phase of the nursing process. The more complete the care plan records, the higher the ordinal score thus obtained, indicating more complete levels of documented systematic care planning for individuals. Each phase of the nursing process can thus achieve a maximum score as follows:

Table 15 Maximum section scores of nursing process phases using documentary analytic checklist

NP PHASE:	MAXIMUM SCORE:
Assessment	51
Planning	36
Implementation	36
Evaluation	45
TOTAL SCORE:	168

Applying this criterion to each care plan under study (f=50), the following results were obtained (see Table 16).

Ward R1

Table 16 R1 Ward Care Plan scores

Nursing Process Phase	Max Section Score	Care Plan number									
		1	2	3	4	5	6	7	8	9	10
Assessment	51	36	36	36	27	35	37	35	35	28	34
Planning	36	20	30	30	25	28	24	21	23	19	13
Implementation	36	34	34	35	30	31	25	35	33	28	30
Evaluation	45	33	36	11	13	36	21	36	28	16	27

Analysis of care plans for R1 ward, whilst showing no maximum section scores, displays highly variant scoring, particularly in the implementation phase. Care Plans 3 and 4 score lowest, both in the evaluation phase; and Care Plans 9 and 10 in the care planning phase. Care plan scores in the assessment phase range from 28 to 37, with a mean score of 33; care planning ranges from 13 to 30, with a mean score of 23; implementation scores range from 25 to 35, with a mean score of 31; and evaluation scores range from 11 to 36, with a mean score of 26.

Ward R2

Table 17 R2 Ward Care Plan scores

Nursing Process Phase	Max Section Score	Care Plan number									
		1	2	3	4	5	6	7	8	9	10
Assessment	51	33	21	35	15	19	43	17	26	24	32
Planning	36	14	9	26	15	16	27	26	24	26	16
Implementation	36	24	17	30	23	22	29	30	20	23	17
Evaluation	45	39	9	30	9	19	27	34	7	32	26

Analysis of R2 ward care plan scores reveals no Care Plans with a maximum section score. Whilst there seem to be a wide variety of care planning skills, Care Plans 2, 4 and 8 score particularly poorly, especially in the evaluation phase. Assessment scores range from 15 to 43, with a mean score of 26; care planning scores range from 9 to 27, with a mean score of 20; implementation scores range from 17 to 30, with a mean score of 23; and evaluation scores range from 7 to 39, with a mean score of 23.

Ward R3

Table 18 R3 Ward Care Plan scores

Nursing Process Phase	Max Section Score	Care Plan number									
		1	2	3	4	5	6	7	8	9	10
Assessment	51	25	34	35	21	23	34	31	31	32	34
Planning	36	19	27	23	22	22	23	26	30	25	22
Implementation	36	30	30	28	28	25	28	31	36	33	28
Evaluation	45	22	28	18	16	5	15	27	28	27	28

Analysis of care plan section scores on R3 ward reveals that only one care plan achieved a maximum possible section score (Care Plan 8, implementation). Other scores vary from relatively high to low indicating a wide degree of care planning skills of nurses within the ward. Assessment scores range from 21 to 34, with a mean score of 30; care planning scores range from 19 to 30, with a mean score of 24, implementation scores range from 25 to 36, with a mean score of 27; and evaluation scores range from 5 to 28, with a mean score of 21. Care Plan 5 is the lowest scoring care plan, with a particularly low score of 5 in the evaluation phase.

Ward E1

Table 19 E1 Ward Care Plan scores

Nursing Process Phase	Max Section Score	Care Plan number									
		1	2	3	4	5	6	7	8	9	10
Assessment	51	38	34	39	38	29	26	25	27	29	27
Planning	36	26	23	23	23	25	23	12	18	22	22
Implementation	36	31	27	32	32	26	31	25	27	29	28
Evaluation	45	34	29	24	28	30	30	32	24	22	29

Analysis of E1 ward care plans again reveals no maximum scores in the care planning as reflected in the documentation. Care planning scores within these data sets appear more consistent, with scores being relatively similar except for Care Plan 7, whose care planning phase scores lower than the others. Assessment scores range from 25 to 39, with a mean score of 31; care planning scores range from 12 to 26, with a mean score of 22; implementation scores range from 25 to 32, with a mean score of 29; and evaluation scores range from 22 to 34, with a mean score of 28.

Ward E2

Table 20 E2 Ward Care Plan scores

Nursing Process Phase	Max Section Score	Care Plan number									
		1	2	3	4	5	6	7	8	9	10
Assessment	51	44	43	51	48	44	50	41	29	42	47
Planning	36	13	30	32	29	28	33	27	9	27	24
Implementation	36	14	23	28	33	29	30	30	15	22	25
Evaluation	45	27	35	39	33	35	43	38	16	21	37

Analysis of care plans on E2 ward again show no maximum care planning scores. However, assessment scores for most care plans are relatively high. Again there is variety of care planning skill levels as indicated, particularly within the low-scoring Care Plans 1 and 8, especially in the care planning, implementation and evaluation phases. Assessment scores range from 29 to 51, with a mean score of 44; care planning scores range from 9 to 33, with a mean score of 25; implementation scores range from 14 to 33, with a mean score of 25; and evaluation scores range from 16 to 43, with a mean score of 32.

Documentary analytic checklist: qualitative findings

Although the care plan scores provide quantitative data which can be used for baseline measures of care and subsequent comparisons after re-measure, it is the qualitative aspects of the analysis that are perhaps the most important. Consideration should be given as to why checklist items score low: hence qualitative interpretations are required if accurate description is desired. For example, documentation may show that an evaluation has not been carried out; but it may be the case that the evaluation date has not yet been reached. Hence although scores may indicate anomalous areas, individual accounts of each item were checked to ensure validity of the low score.

Detailed analysis of each of the documentary audits revealed numerous practices that could be modified, improving nursing skills and thus influencing the quality of care given to patients. However, for purposes of this report, descriptive comments are confined to those individual items that have scored zero (0) consistently within the five locations. As can be seen from Tables 16 to 20, patterns of low-scoring in similar categories emerge. The following descriptive details of "anomalous" areas in care planning are common to all five locations: that is, they occur both internally and externally to Rampton Hospital.

General deficits in assessment phase

Frequently patients' problems were not listed but were evident within assessment documents, although they required teasing out. Where problems were listed they lacked any detail, often being stated as single, unrelated comments.

Records concerning reasons for admission were often excluded from assessments. This resulted in the absence of potentially vital information relating to the patient's problem. If reasons for admission are being omitted from assessment then it is unlikely that care plans will relate to this important problem area.

Where patients' problems had been identified there was little evidence of these being prioritised. If problems are tackled simply in an ad hoc fashion, care planning will never effectively address them. Implementation of related patient care without due attention to clinical and social priorities could call into

114

question the validity or relevance of the associated care plan.

Whilst patients were clearly involved to some degree with self assessment, there was little substantive evidence of discussions taking place with patients about their problems. Whilst recognising that not all mentally ill patients are well enough to participate to any great degree, it is essential that they should be involved in determining elements of their care. The validity of these and other contributions are then available for discussion within the ward team.

General deficits in care planning phase

Incentives and reinforcers were rarely offered to patients within their care plan. If patients are to respond to care planning then it would appear desirable that some appropriate reward system is offered. Patients are much more likely to respond if they receive symbolic recognition of their achievements, either in terms of token or other economies, or in the form of social reinforcement.

Few care plans reflected collaboration in care between nurses and members of other care disciplines. Despite the fact that patients are out of ward environment for up to two-thirds of the waking day, no evidence was found of extra-ward continuity of care planning. To some degree this lack of continuity is bound to vitiate care plans which rely on shared goals and consistency of treatment between hospital departments.

Similarly, multidisciplinary care staff were rarely involved in the planning of care for patients. Only one ward held regular discussions which included non-nursing members of related care disciplines; but even then they were seldom involved in systematic collaboration to achieve continuity of care.

Whilst some patients were involved in their assessments, few were actually involved in discussions about the actual structure of their resultant care plan. Consequently, some goal-setting appeared unrealistic, both in terms of manageable progress steps and in terms of declared final outcomes. Where patients were so involved, goals appeared to be much more achievable; and the documents supported this.

General deficits in implementation phase

Intershift communication in the two external ward contexts generally appeared "hit-and-miss". Certainly within some care plans and related documentation, intershift communication was detected; but it was still considerably lacking in others. Significantly, within internal ward contexts little evidence of any intershift communication could be found. In particular, shift changeovers were noted to contain no relevant information that could recognisably reflect care planning for patients.

Whilst reflecting care related to the care plan in some cases, progress reports were often misleading and generalised. For example: "Tom had a good day". Progress reports largely did not reflect the actual care given; but instead offered a somewhat uninformative general statement. In addition progress notes were difficult to read; and, in the case of multiple care plans, it was often difficult to recognise which notes belonged to which care plan.

Although some care plans had prioritised care problems within the assessment hierarchy, resultant care was seldom delivered in priority order, making the assessed care priorities largely meaningless from a therapeutic point of view.

General deficits in evaluation phase

There was little evidence of ongoing assessment between evaluation dates. This meant that in some cases "desirable" patient behaviours were clearly occurring more frequently; but with delayed modifications in the care plan.
In some cases these modifications were left for several weeks until formal evaluation dates.

In several cases across all locations evaluations were carried out on dates that did not correspond with those set out in the care plan.

Internal and external contexts: broad comparisons

The data suggest that there is wide variance in nurses' care planning skills throughout both internal and external locations. Some nurses appear significantly more proficient than others; and most care plans reflect differing problems. Quite clearly the episodic educational preparation for nursing process identified within the pilot (Robinson, 1988) has resulted in relatively few nurses being able to carry out the components of care planning with any degree of competency. However, if one "pools" existing nursing knowledge, most, if not all, of the requisite skills seem to be present; and a rationalisation and "pulling together" of these skills could substantially improve care planning for patients.

Regarding internal locations, nursing staff located on R1, R2 and R3 wards display more skills related to the implementation phase than to any other phase. This evidence supports the view that nurses have tended to be "doers" rather than "thinkers"; and have not yet come to terms with the advantages of systematic recording of care details.

The external locations appear to display slightly different deficits. For example, in E2 ward, there appear to be greater strengths in the assessment and evaluation areas; with deficits in care planning and implementation. In the case of this ward, there appears to be an imbalance towards paperwork rather than care intervention. Regarding E1 ward, here there appears to be stronger emphasis on intervention; with care planning, and especially assessment, being considerably weaker areas.

7 Patient interview findings

The following patient interview findings are presented in similar thematic order for ease of comparison. There are no patient findings for R1 ward. Despite attempts to interview members of the R1 sub-sample, it was felt that responses on this ward were invalidated due to severe mental impairment of informants, which results in distorted and often irrelevant information.

Internal wards (R2 AND R3)

Recreational interests and interaction

Most informants (sixteen) said that interactions with nurses were beneficial and worthwhile. Relationships with nursing staff were particularly enjoyable when participating in wards events such as snooker, cards or board games. Only two informants had no interest and preferred to be on their own. The others felt that they were unsure as to the value of recreational interests and preferred to be left alone. Five of the informants felt that there was not enough variety on offer in terms of recreational facilities, feeling that as a result of this they became bored rather quickly.

Nurse-patient relationship

Seventeen informants felt that there were always nursing staff available if they required to contact or talk to them. Only one informant felt that nursing staff were not always available. Feeling amongst patients was divided in that half felt there was no key person to whom they could relate; whilst the other half felt their key nurse was always available to talk to them. In the former group, some patients felt that relationships with the key nurse were artificially forced.

Nurse-patient communication

Informants felt that nursing staff mostly had time to talk to patients; and nurses would sit and chat to them. Topics included both general daily events and structured discussions. However, there was a feeling that, although nurses have time to chat, it is perhaps only when *they* want to do so. Again the consensus of informants was that they had never been rejected, particularly in relation to key workers.

Patient involvement in care planning

Almost all informants (sixteen) mentioned that nurses discussed their care plans with them and that they were involved in deciding relevant parts of their care, some describing care plans in detail. Again the same informants felt that they were included in most aspects of care planning; and could describe quite accurately their discussions in formulating the care plans. Only one informant felt that care decisions should be left to staff.

Direct care

Nine informants felt that nurses were giving input to their current care problems and that nurses were helping them. All of these informants were able to talk with confidence about the areas of care that they were receiving. In addition it was felt that care input was being given on a regular basis and that the patients were benefiting from the input. The remaining informants felt that they could not see what nursing staff were doing for them, apart from encouragement to improve their personal appearance; and therefore could not relate to implementation of their care plan.

Social contact

In spite of the national catchment served by Rampton Hospital, only one informant felt that he was isolated and that no external visitors came to see him because of the distance. The remainder (nineteen) received visits during most weeks; and spoke of the importance of family contact facilities and the communication links between family and nursing staff.

External wards (E1 AND E2)

Recreational interests and interaction

Almost all informants (eighteen) felt that there were more than adequate opportunities for interaction and recreational interests with staff. All informants again felt that most nurses joined in the various recreational activities, but in particular key nurses gave the most input. Six informants criticised the lack of facilities, often referring to them as repetitive and boring.

Nurse-patient relationship

Most informants (sixteen) felt that there was always someone about that they could turn to for assistance. It was felt that there was always someone to talk to, even if it was not a key nurse. Whilst generally recognising that there were certain staff who were assigned to them as key nurses, they tended to have relationships with most of the ward staff. Three informants felt that their key nurse spent more time with others, indicating that s/he was not always available.

Nurse-patient communication

All informants felt that, although some key nurses may be involved with other patients, there was always a member of staff to talk to if they wished. Similarly, when approached by patients, staff members always had time for conversation. Conversation differed according to the patient; and ranged from communications about visits to the discussion of care programmes. Only two patients felt that there were a minority of staff who did not have as much time for them as they would have liked.

Patient involvement in care planning

Fifteen informants felt that much time was spent by ward staff and doctors in discussing and planning their care. Most could remember details of their care; but could not relate it to care planning. Clearly with these informants there was much evidence of discussion taking place. Five informants knew that the nurses were doing "something" for them; but could not recall any discussions taking place. Two informants did specifically mention that they would prefer the care staff to decide their care programmes for them; and were not bothered about personal involvement.

Direct care

Six informants had some insight into the areas that nurses were helping them with. In particular, it was felt that nurses were helping patients with their anxieties, and helping them to "cope". These informants also suggested that they were satisfied with the care received from nurses: and that nurses were tackling the important care issues necessary to help them get well.

Twelve patients were unsure as to precisely how they were being helped; but stressed their regular contact with staff. Three patients felt that nurses were not particularly helpful at the present time; and generally did not bother with them.

Social contact

All but one informant felt that there were no problems regarding social contact, although visiting times could be more flexible. Similarly, informants felt that there were more than adequate opportunities for families and friends to visit them. It was felt that these visits - especially those by a spouse - were of enormous value in helping with the relief of anxieties. In addition it was felt that staff encourage relatives to visit patients.

Discussion

The findings in the four wards (R2, R3, E1 and E2) reveal similarities which are particularly important from the consumer viewpoint, and especially in terms of consumer satisfaction.

Generally, patients in both internal and external locations felt that there were ample opportunities for social interaction with nursing staff. Despite having some recreational facilities within the ward, there was a general feeling that these were "lacking". This was especially important since the lack of facilities often led to frustration, and in some cases to anxiety.

Most patients in all locations felt that they had good relationships with staff; but these tended to be with key workers. This was especially interesting, since some patients felt that this artificial "forcing" of nurses to work with them was not as therapeutic as if patients themselves were involved in helping to choose their own key workers. It was felt that quite often nurse-patient relationships were consequently somewhat restricted and limited to relatively few staff.

Despite occasional limitations in gaining access to key workers, patients found that there was "always someone available" who would listen and talk to them. According to the patients, only one ward at Rampton Hospital showed appreciable levels of patient involvement in individual care planning.

Remarkably, these patients tended to be able to describe their planned care in considerable detail. Quite obviously, given the opportunity, most patients have a valid contribution to make through involvement in determining their own care programmes.

Similarly, the involvement of the consumer is much more likely to develop authentic relationships and promote health care. Patients on other wards, whilst recognising that they were involved in "discussions" surrounding their care, were unsure as to what this consisted of; and sometimes equated it with group work. Regarding social contact, there was a consensus within all locations that patients were receiving adequate visits from relatives and families. These were thought of as being especially valuable and therapeutic by patients.

The patient interview data clearly show that, given appropriate opportunities, the majority of patients want to be part of decision-making within the care processes. Nurses now need to make substantial changes in quality procedures, aimed at bringing the consumer further to the fore in the care and treatment debate.

8 Nurse interview findings

The following nurse interview findings are presented in similar order to that of the patient findings (i.e. data on internal locations followed by data on external locations).

Internal ward findings (Wards R1, R2 and R3)

Introduction to the nursing process

Five nurse informants had trained more recently than the original introduction of the nursing process at Rampton Hospital in 1981. Thus their first introduction to nursing process was in their nurse training in which it formed part of the 1982 Syllabus. Four nurses stated that it was the nursing process coordinators who first made them aware of it.

Nineteen nurse informants stated that insufficient care and thought went into planning and implementation of the nursing process. For most "it just appeared, and we were told to get on with it by senior managers"!

Four nurses had attended the Open University course on Systematic Approaches to Care (OU P553); and felt that it was relevant to some degree, though it did not relate to the specific needs of forensic psychiatric nurses. It was generally felt that the nursing process was "coming, so get on with it!

This had clearly resulted in the nurses who had been introduced to the nursing process at ward level feeling that this was a large task to undertake with little or no support. Accompanying perceptions included the classical response, "more paperwork"; and "suddenly we had to put twenty-five patients on it"!

Advantages of the nursing process

The majority of nurse informants (nineteen) were in no doubt that the nursing process had clear advantages that far outweighed its disadvantages. Even nurse informants who were sceptical concerning the manner of its introduction saw its potential benefit for patients. Advantages that were mentioned most frequently were: "the provision of continuity of care"; "it gives clear directions for care"; "it allows patients to participate in their own care programmes"; and "it allows both patients and staff to be more informed". By far the most frequently mentioned advantage was that it facilitates consistency in care.

Perceived disadvantages were few, but were equally important to staff. These consisted of the time involved in completing the care plan paperwork; and the lack of multidisciplinary input: that is, it is considered to be the *nursing* process rather than implying involvement of other disciplines. Others (eight) felt that in certain situations there was "too much" nursing process; and felt that other aspects of care were perhaps neglected.

Structure of the nursing care plan

Table 21 shows the stages of the nursing process and traces informants' familiarity with the four phases. All but twelve nurse informants were able to describe the four phases, displaying a good basic knowledge (see Table 21 on next page).

Table 21 Wards R1, R2 and R3 : Nurses' identification of nursing process phases (N = 30)

Nurse	Assessment	Planning	Implementation	Evaluation
1	A	P	I	E
2	A	P	I	E
3	A	P	I	E
4	A	P	I	E
5	A	-	I	-
6	A	P	-	E
7	A	P	I	E
8	A	-	-	-
9	A	P	I	E
10	A	P	-	E
11	A	A	I	E
12	A	P	I	E
13	A	P	I	E
14	A	P	I	E
15	A	P	I	E
16	A	P	I	E
17	A	P	I	E
18	A	-	-	E
19	A	P	-	-
20	A	P	I	-
21	A	P	I	E
22	A	P	-	E
23	A	P	-	E
24	A	P	-	E
25	A	P	I	E
26	A	P	I	E
27	-	P	I	E
28	A	P	I	E
29	A	P	-	E
30	A	P	I	E

Defining the nursing process

Although some definitions of the nursing process were much briefer than others, there was no doubt that all nurse informants could indicate the main points. Whilst there were several styles of definition, all contained the "key" elements of contemporary definitions: that is, "individualised", "systematic", "prioritised needs", "assessment", "planning", "implementation" and "evaluation".

Practical outcomes of the nursing process

All nurse informants (thirty) felt that care planning actually affected patient care on their ward. Throughout there was a consensus that, by using care planning, it was possible to help patients improve their current health status and/or skills. In particular informants stated that progress of patients could be seen particularly when evaluating the written care plans.

As a result nurses could actually observe the improvements. Other informants stated how care planning not only helped patient care but enhanced staff/patient relationships and the professional development of nurses.

Communicating the care plan

All nurses felt that communication had improved since introduction of the nursing process. They felt that there was a variety of possible methods for communicating the patients' care plans; although there were some differences of opinion as to who should do it. Some informants (five) felt that all nurses should have responsibility for communication; whilst others (eight) felt that the key nurse should be the person centrally involved.

Prior to the advent of care plans there had been little or no communication about problems of individual patients. In order to ensure that all members of the team were familiar with them, several methods were used. These included: regular ward meetings to discuss care plans; verbal communication together with written notes on all new care plans, inviting inter-shift comments; ward meetings; ward rounds; and case conferences.

Multidisciplinary involvement in care planning

Nurse informants were divided as to who should have responsibility for input to care planning. Firstly, it was felt that the care plan was a *nursing* care plan to be used by nurses. Here, other disciplines should formulate their own. However, it was felt that members of other disciplines could be involved if nurses felt they were needed.

By contrast, others felt that, whilst multidisciplinary working had started, there should be more multidisciplinary involvement in care planning. It was felt that the other disciplines should contribute as appropriate to the care plan. This indicated a belief that various health disciplines should bring their specialist skills to assist to give a more holistic approach.

Monitoring care

All nurse informants (thirty) expressed the view that there is a need continuously to monitor the nursing process. It was recognised that there had been no monitoring since the nursing process coordinators completed their time in post during the latter half of 1986. It was clear that nurse informants were still reflecting rather angrily on the lack of support they felt they had experienced in initiating the nursing process, particularly from the Staff Education Centre. It was generally felt that documentation should be continuously monitored; especially since, in many instances, it was not being done properly.

There was a variety of opinions on who should actually carry out this monitoring; with the following main nominees: nurse specialist; ward sister or charge nurse; unit manager; and the quality assurance department. These latter comments reflect that nurse informants were generally convinced that care planning could influence an improved *quality* of life for patients through its implementation; and, by the introduction of some systematic monitoring, shortfalls could be addressed. This it was felt would result in improved skills development for staff and improved quality of life for patients.

External ward findings (Wards E1 and E2)

Introduction to the nursing process

Half nurse informants (ten) felt that they had received no original introduction to the nursing process. Generally it had been expected of them simply to get on with it. The feelings associated with this were that little support was offered, despite a clear need and request from staff. The only support that was made available was given by those few members of nursing staff who were fortunate enough to attend seminars or meetings on the nursing process.

The remaining nurse informants, stated that they had been introduced to the nursing process through training or a briefing letter explaining its implementation, followed up by short seminars and workshops. In addition the educational input was thought to be lacking, with little or no follow-up afterwards.

Advantages of the nursing process

Most (seventeen) nurse informants felt that there were clear advantages in the nursing process, although there were also some key disadvantages. Main disadvantages included the extensive paperwork, which seemed to grow as some nursing staff became more familiar with the concept. As the initial model was adapted to suit individual ward and patient requirements, the paperwork seemed to double in size.

Advantages were clearly recognised; with informants frequently talking about the effect which the nursing process had on patients. It was felt that, by individualising care, nurses were working more together with common views and goals in mind and that it helped nurses think more systematically.

Structure of the nursing care plan

As can be seen from Table 22 there appeared to be a wide variance in care planning skills within the external sample; indicating that over half (fourteen) of the nurse informants could not identify the four phases of the nursing process. Three nurses (numbers nine, eleven and twelve in Table 22) could not give any clear interpretation of *any* of the four phases.

Nurse	Assessment	Planning	Implementation	Evaluation
1	A	P	I	E
2	A	P	-	E
3	A	-	I	-
4	A	P	I	-
5	-	P	I	E
6	A	P	-	E
7	A	P	I	E
8	A	P	I	E
9	-	-	-	-
10	A	P	I	E
11	-	-	-	-
12	-	-	-	-
13	A	P	-	-
14	A	P	-	-
15	A	-	-	E
16	A	P	-	E
17	A	P	-	-
18	A	-	-	E
19	A	P	I	E
20	A	P	I	E

Defining the nursing process

Twelve nurse informants were able to define the nursing process within the
current and varied definitions that exist. These nurses were able to give key
phrases and definitions that are associated with the nursing process, such as
"systematic care for patients"; "individualising"; "determining patients'
problems"; and "setting objectives for patients and staff to work to".

The remaining nurse informants (eight) were unable to give any accurate
account that could be related to the nursing process. However, most indicated
that it was a method for actually improving care in some way.

Practical outcomes of the nursing process

Fifteen nurse informants felt that the nursing process did have some practical outcome although some were unsure as to how this was. Nurses felt that it was a tool to enable patients' problems to be identified and actioned. By monitoring the implementation of care, it was possible in some cases to see that patients were actually progressing. Six nurses felt that there was nothing better than the nursing process for measuring patient outcomes. Outcomes were felt to be an important part of maintaining standards of care that are reflective of patient needs.

Some of the remaining nurse informants (three) felt that it was sometimes difficult to state whether patients actually benefited from care planning; or whether their improvement was really attributable to the general care given. This was because they felt that they were not always involved in care planning; and were unsure as to its effectiveness.

Communicating the care plan

Most nurse informants had mixed views about the communicative value of care plans. However, all nurse informants said that care plans were communicated to some degree at shift handover; but that this was sometimes limited to only a few nurses, usually the most senior qualified nurses. However, it was felt that the care plan is there for people to read and familiarise themselves with the care that required to be given. In addition, seven nurses spoke about improved communication because the care plan improved continuity of care through oral and written accounts.

Two nurse informants suggested that, despite the information being available to be communicated, it was left to the individual to be informed. This was supported by their comments that there was often not enough time to read care notes, as they were always given duties to perform.

Multidisciplinary involvement in care planning

Most nurse informants (eleven) felt that there should be some involvement by members of other care disciplines in care planning for patients. Seven informants felt that there were few times when other disciplines were involved in care planning for patients. Three nurses felt that members of other care disciplines should be involved with care planning; but only if the patient went into their department for therapeutic intervention.

These nurses tended to imply that the nursing process was really about *nursing* interventions rather than about other disciplines being involved. Again, two nursing auxiliaries felt that they did not really have any views on multidisciplinary involvement; but realised its potential advantages.

Monitoring care

Most nurse informants (nineteen) felt that the nursing process should be monitored if the quality of service was continually to improve. It was felt that there had been a general lack of support throughout its introduction and implementation. it was thought that, if some form of monitoring were in place, this would result in providing education in which more knowledge and related skills could be gained. One charge nurse felt that it was already being monitored by himself on a regular basis; but little evidence was forthcoming from the rest of the ward nurse informants to suggest any advantages accruing from this. There was, however, no doubt among these nurses that some form of monitoring could lead to the improvement of nurses' skills and lead to an improved quality of life for patients.

Similar perceptions in the five locations

Few nurse informants within the five locations felt that they had received adequate support when the nursing process was first introduced. Similarly, most felt that the nursing process "just appeared", rather than being systematically introduced. Frequently it appeared that nurse managers within the five locations had sent nursing process packages to wards with little or no other support, expecting, in some cases, all patients to be put on care plans, often with unrealistic deadlines. Whilst there appears to have been a lack of relevant education for all nurses, nursing auxiliaries appear to be the main staff who have lacked such programmes.

Advantages of the nursing process were seen as far outweighing its potential disadvantages, in terms of patient improvement and communication. It was seen that the nursing process provided a clear framework within which to improve staff skills; patients' quality of life; and bring about more effective inter-shift communication. This, it was felt, would help nursing staff focus more on patients' individual problems and outcomes. The bulky and complicated paperwork often implemented appears to be the main disadvantage across the samples.

There was a clear lack of ability by most nurse informants within the five locations to recall or define all four stages of the nursing process. This reflects back to the original, haphazard implementation and lack of educational support. Most nurses were able to offer a brief definition of the nursing process; but this tended to be couched in a series of key words and phrases, rather than as a short, simple definition. One ward in an external location seemed to lack in this area more than wards in the other four locations. Again this tended to affect nursing auxiliaries more than other nurses.

Nurse informants in all locations were virtually unanimous that care planning helped improve the health status of patients; despite their occasionally seeming unable to discuss in detail what it actually was. Many nurse informants referred to the improvements reflected in the documentation as providing evidence. Informants in all locations felt that care planning did influence communication positively in the patients' favour, with few exceptions. it was thought to be a way of getting people to discuss individual care, as well as providing visual evidence for others' reference.

Multidisciplinary involvement in care was supported by nurse informants in most of the locations. Each reflected that there were clear advantages about involving other disciplines in care planning. However, some nurses were keen to stipulate that members of other disciplines should only be involved if patients were involved in their areas. Similarly, nurse informants in each location spoke about the positive effects that monitoring the nursing process could have. Generally, it was felt that this could help improve staff knowledge and related skills, as well as helping improve the quality of life for patients.

9 Discussion

Theoretical retrospect: relationship of theory to study findings

Initially it is appropriate to examine in more general terms the extent to which data obtained in the present study bear on the theoretical issues discussed in Chapter One.

General retrospect

The pilot study (Robinson, 1988, 1990 and 1990a) helped clarify the fundamental links between nursing process and quality care; especially important since consumers increasingly demand quality with individual care (see, for example, Department of Health, 1989b).

The need for nurses to develop a problem solving approach to professional activity (Lamonica, 1979; Hunt, 1985) was well illustrated in the attitudes of nurses. The resultant nursing process, whilst concerned with transforming nursing into a research-based activity reliant upon empirical evaluation (Aggleton and Chalmers, 1986) did not represent systematic use of the four stages of the nursing process (Hurst, 1987).

Frequently nurses were unable to describe all the stages (assessment, care planning, implementation and evaluation) necessary to carry out systematic care planning (Sheehan, 1991), frequently missing key components. This was an issue represented within anomalous areas of the documentary analysis and through the infrequent delivery of individualised care represented within ward-based observations.

The principal advantage of the nursing process, its encouragement of more systematic assessment of the patient's condition (Mayers, 1983; Hardy, 1987) was apparent to some degree from the documentary analysis; though there is much to be improved here. Nurses frequently spoke about the advantages of the introduction of individualised care, including more effective care delivery and patient involvement, delivered through the nursing process (Kitson, 1986).

The view that the introduction was flawed with problems by nurses being "left to get on with it" (Hayward, 1986; Robinson, 1990) was repeatedly voiced by nursing staff. This finding must also be seen in relation to the keen awareness of nurses of the existence of specific deficits in their knowledge and skills necessary for effective care planning (Sheehan, 1991).

The conviction that "nurses were told to get on with it" (De La Cuesta, 1983; Robinson, 1990a) serves to support their perception that, whilst there was some emphasis on education and training, little staff support was offered at grass roots level (De La Cuesta, 1983). Similarly, informants felt that the nursing process "just appeared", rather than being introduced through a normative-reeducative approach (Ashworth, 1985).

Advantages of the nursing process perceived by nursing staff appeared to outweigh disadvantages. Even though scepticism existed, much benefit was seen from patients' participation in care programmes (Baines, 1981). This was a view also supported by patient informants, who felt "more involved" with their care programmes, some describing them in considerable detail.

Time-consuming exercises, and especially increased paperwork, have been frequently identified as problematic (Hayward, 1986); resulting in nurses seeing the nursing process as "just a paper exercise". Whilst nurses support this, sometimes their knowledge base appears weak; and remedies remain within re-education strategies (Ashworth, 1985). Regarding documentary evidence, generalised notes and poor record-keeping reflected these views; as did low levels of assessment and care planning within ward observations.

The apparent difficulties of nurses in psychiatric settings to define their role, and related difficulties in rehabilitating patients without a clear perception of their role, has resulted in attempts still being made to fit the patient into traditional institutional care regimes (Mackie and Welch, 1982; Barrowclough et al, 1984; Whyte and Youhill, 1984; Robinson, 1990 and 1990a).

Lack of understanding of the underlying principles of nursing process is demonstrated by nurses' lack of perceptions of systematic care delivery (Hurst, 1987); anomalous care planning within the documentary analysis; and a lack of individual care and direct contact with patients in ward-based observations, resulting in (albeit unconscious) depersonalised care regimes (Kitson, 1986).

Whilst nursing is concerned with enabling the individual to achieve and maintain optimal physical and social wellbeing (Department of Health, 1993b), patients have often been excluded from decision-making within care programmes (Liddle and Gilby, 1991). Patient informants reported being involved to some degree, although such involvement was thought in some instances to be "artificial". The commonly-held view that the patient is "too ill" to be asked about care programmes (Green, 1987; Donabedian, 1993) was to some extent evident in the responses both of patient and staff informants. Observational evidence offered less support. The interview findings thus tend to support the notion that involving patients as consumers in care is still an "add-on", rather than part of everyday care (Pringle, 1992).

The last decade has seen a considerable shift in emphasis from a task-oriented approach to nursing to one based upon individualised care (Sheehan, 1991) However, there is some way to go to influence successful change. Individual care has become central to the values of nursing (Reed, 1993); but much remains to be done to sustain impact at grass roots level.

Although nurse researchers and tutors to some degree responded to the challenge of the introduction of individualised care programmes (Alexander, 1980; Pearson, 1986; Brooking, 1988) and contributed to its understanding, few if any contributed to its everyday working concepts. This proposition is supported by nurses' comments and especially by the low levels of individualised care reflected within ward-based observations. However, where research-based activities have been used to facilitate related educational change (for example, Carton, 1990) significant increase in nursing process behaviours has been reflected within the ward-based observations.

Akinsanya (1986) expresses the need for a reappraisal of preparation for nurse educators, which must have some influence on the status of implementation of individualised care programmes. Owing to lack of understanding, implementation and identification of skills deficits displayed by informants, it is essential that teachers are prepared adequately (Sheehan, 1989). Therefore programmes seeking to implement such concepts as the nursing process need to involve not only teachers but researchers and students who, through empirical investigation, would continue to restructure their views of knowledge (Driver and Erickson, 1983).

The need to implement change in a carefully-phased, normative-reeducative manner (Ashworth, 1985) and the need for repeated systematic enquiry into its implementation (Hayward, 1986) are well-supported within the nursing comments. Failure to implement successfully will only mean a lack of quality care for patients.

Implications of Leininger's care constructs

It is anticipated that empirical studies such as the present one, offering a multi-method approach, can contribute significantly to such change. The use of more than one method in a study (for example, observational techniques combined with documentary analysis and questioning) more accurately to depict the phenomenon being investigated (Denzin, 1970; Cowman, 1993) may serve to validate emergent theory.

The development of appropriate care indicators through detailed observations of nursing activity drew substantially on qualitative and quantitative methodology. This was used as a theoretical base to discover the nature and essence of forensic psychiatric care. Such methods have been described as meaningful and refreshing in their discovery of human nature (Leininger, 1992). Leininger (1985) also avers that people are not reducible to measurable objects; and that therefore qualitative accounts are particularly useful. Thus, whilst accepting the differences between the two methods, neither method should be exclusive of the other; and when brought together, as within this study, they may start to provide a richness in the understanding of human beings (Cowman, 1993).

The importance of observation in discovering first-hand what nurses do needs to be stressed (Akinsanya, 1986). Using descriptive observational techniques initially used by King, Raynes and Tizard, (1971) and by Reed (1978), observations were categorised into meaningful constructs, using a "grounded theory" approach (see, for example, Baker et al, 1992). Core constructs were identified and piloted in earlier research (Robinson, 1987, 1988) in contexts that related both to forensic and mainstream psychiatric care.

Contemporary anthropological researchers stress the need for investigators to obtain qualitative, documented, descriptive accounts of observed and verified behaviour revealing the essence, nature and processes of a culture (Leininger, 1981). Questioning of informants gives a differing perspective in supporting observational data. The descriptions of staff and patients generate rich material that can be compared and contrasted with that obtained by other methods (Carter, 1985; Davis, 1984). Examination of life situations in which staff and patients find themselves has been particularly useful within the nursing and patient interviews in the present study (see also Lynch-Sauer, 1985).

The conceptual theory-generating model developed by Leininger (1986) identifies twenty-seven caring constructs and was used as a basis in the present study to generate and test hypotheses and methods. The constructs are identified in Table 23 (see next page).

Table 23 Leininger's conceptual theory-generating model: care constructs (after Leininger, 1986)

1	comfort	14	nurturance
2	compassion	15	presence
3	concern	16	protection
4	coping	17	restoration
5	empathy	18	sharing
6	enabling	19	stimulating
7	facilitating	20	stress alleviation
8	interest	21	succouring
9	involvement	22	support
10	health consultation	23	surveillance
11	health maintenance	24	tenderness
12	helping	25	touching
13	love	26	trust

(each of these constructs has many sub-descriptions)

These care constructs were derived as the result of anthropological studies enabling "grounded theory" techniques to identify appropriate concepts which represent the area under study. When categorised they enable a "socially meaningful" interpretation of interactions and events that enable health professionals to interpret the process of intervention (Meichenbaum, 1977).

Dissatisfaction with quality indicators

The lack of coherence of the general body of quality studies, which rarely build on one another (Shaw, 1988) supports the notion that continuous adaptation of existing methods for use in different health care settings may have a salutary effect (Shaw, 1988).

In the constantly changing world of contemporary health care, such "static" criteria are bound to fail (Ellis, 1987). It is suggested that one reason for the literature highlighting current deficits within quality methods is this tendency to lack of review and modification (see, for example, Smith, 1986; Dickson, 1987; Redfern and Norman, 1990; Balogh, 1991; Oliver and West, 1991). The present study seeks to move forward by adapting and innovating methods as well as developing dynamic changes within care constructs.

A key motivation for the present study is that within the Special Hospitals no researcher had as yet attempted systematically to describe nursing care; and therefore little if any research material could be drawn upon. However, substantial material was available from the general context of psychiatric nursing which has been of considerable use.

Carers and consumers of care increasingly demand quality of care linked to individualised care (Department of Health, 1989a). Paradoxically, recent quality audits show some evidence of individualised care being treated as a paper exercise (Hurst and Dean, 1987). This finding is well supported by data from the documentary analysis in the present study, especially with regard to the production of generalised, non-specific nursing reports.

The literature on nursing process stresses the uniqueness of the patient and the importance of focusing care around his/her discrete needs, or around the problems of the individual (Henderson, 1982). Integration of individual care within the concept of quality is evident within many audit instruments: for example, Psychiatric Audit (Hurst, 1988); Nursing Process Management Scale (Brooking, 1986); and Monitor (Goldstone, 1987). Lian (1985) describes nursing process as being the fundamental step towards quality assurance. Whilst differing concepts of quality exist, the individual patient remains at the centre of the quality debate.

Both in the present study and its pilot (Robinson 1988) it is argued that, if patients are not getting the required interventions identified within care plans, then their quality of life and health care must be less than optimal. The Strategy for Nursing (Department of Health, 1989b) clearly states that "... patients have a right to receive the best possible care" (see also Department of Health, 1989ac, 1991, 1992, 1993ab).

Evidence presented so far in this study reinforces the existence of deficits in individual care delivery which, if overcome, could have a substantial impact on improving quality care to patients, as well as contributing towards staff motivation, skills improvement and job satisfaction (Moores, 1993). Whilst the notion of individualised care has been current for well over a decade, the nursing profession still has to come to grips with the fundamental issue of problem solving through models such as the nursing process (Hurst, 1987; Tanner, 1987).

This requirement is further reinforced by recent governmental statements emphasising a need to ensure that "... there are systems in place to encourage and facilitate development of individualised patient care" (Department of Health, 1993b). Such statements imply that implementation of nursing process has yet to occur in many areas of the National Health Service. Where it is implemented, it still requires much monitoring to become more effective; a view shared by nursing informants in all locations in the present study (see also Hayward ed, 1986).

The last decade has seen an increase in methods designed to evaluate various aspects of service delivery (Goldstone, 1987; Hurst, 1988), though marred by a certain lack of developmental coherence and continuity. Whilst recognising the important contribution of various previous studies of quality, the present study has sought to supply some well-documented shortcomings. Similarly, it has offered a flexible development of care constructs through the use of Leininger's (1986) theory-generating model (see tables 24 and 25 above).

Issues in psychiatric settings

Psychiatric nurses have been accused in the past of being doers rather than thinkers (Thompson, 1979). Evidence regarding nurses' ability to describe the problem-solving approach to the nursing process certainly highlights difficulties, especially within the external locations (see also Hurst, 1987; Hurst and Dean, 1987; Tanner, 1987).

In many health care contexts a shortage of provision for appropriate education has resulted in many nurses never receiving formal education in the concepts of the nursing process (Milne and Turton, 1986). This is reflected in the attitudes of nursing staff within both internal and external locations of the present study, as well as in performance levels of actually carrying out nursing process within the ward-based observations.

Within the context of forensic and mainstream psychiatric nursing, where psychological needs and problems are frequently paramount, it is easy for staff to become over-protective and custodial; and nurses may inadvertently revert back to task-oriented, institutional routines (Barrowclough et al, 1984; Willard, 1984). Low levels of individualised care seen in ward-based observations support the continued existence of these outdated care practices, with some nursing staff obviously unsure what to do with patients. This in turn frequently reflects the lack of planning within ward-based programmes of care.

The added implications in forensic psychiatric care, where patients may be dangerous to themselves or others, means that high levels of security are required within a therapeutic environment (SHSA, 1991). There are several indications within the study that, in the dichotomy between security requirements and individual care, the latter is "losing out" to the former to a considerable degree. Such empirical investigation is necessary if we are to define and understand the nature and context of these care processes (Bowman, 1983; Ashworth, 1985).

Certainly nurses have experienced difficulty in putting care plans into effect;

and considerable time is spent in static supervisory roles, where nurses frequently wait for incidents to happen, rather than adopting a more proactive approach through the use of systematic care planning.

Evidence within some psychiatric contexts suggests that nurses spend approximately two and a half times as long in the ward office as in direct care to patients (Cormack, 1976; Street, 1982; Hurst, 1987, 1993). Observational findings support this view. Both internal and external locations revealed that almost twice as much time was spent in indirect care to patients (up to sixty-eight per cent). Direct care to patients only accounted for approximately twenty eight per cent with little variation in any location. Such low levels of direct care to patients must place theoretical stress on the concept of nursing process (Robinson, 1988) since individual care is extremely low in comparison with other care types.

Nursing process behaviours accounted for between twelve and twenty percent of ward observations. It is worth noting here that in the case of R2 ward (20 per cent NP behaviours), a steady increase was noted in nursing process activity which was attributable to a ward-based teaching programme (Carton, 1990). This increase has been identified within Figure 5 and must illustrate the importance of appropriate measured introduction and training (Sheehan, 1989, 1991; Proctor, 1993).

The burden of administrative duties on the ward charge nurses and other qualified nurses has been considerable (Cormack, 1976); and was well represented within the qualitative analysis of ward observations. Qualified nurses spent considerable time performing varied administrative duties, frequently within office areas, a finding not dissimilar to that of Street (1982). Similarly, charges nurses' infrequent interaction with patients (Cormack, 1983) was well represented within all study locations. This lack of input from qualified nurses serves to emphasise the need for a reappraisal of nursing skills and their appropriate use (Sheehan, 1982; Mitchell, 1984; Akinsanya, 1986). If nurses do not grasp research-based findings in this respect, then their role and ability as providers of quality health care are clearly under threat.

Also noted within Cormack's (1983) study was nursing verbal interaction, which then accounted for some thirteen per cent of staff time. Individualised care centres around communication and the involvement of patients. Observational data reflect current language use by nurses; and illustrate the infrequent verbal contact with patients, although patient interview data reveal their need and desire for "someone to talk to". In support of this, patient relationships with nursing staff require much work, since patient-initiated interactions were considerably low.

Figure 11 highlights the need for a more even balance in relationships, thus increasing individualised care and the therapeutic value it reflects. External

140

locations reflected more verbal interaction than did internal locations. It is not known formally why this might be so; but intuitive reactions suggest more dialogue occurs with patients in external care locations due to the perceived less "dangerous" health state of the patients concerned.

Finally, Hurst and Howard (1988) within an audit programme showed details of direct care to patients which accounted for approximately twenty- five percent of observations; with individual care accounting for less. Observational findings within all locations support low levels of interactions with patients. Within the current findings a pattern of unchanged activity in certain behavioural categories over the last decade has emerged.

Relationship between current and previous findings

Observational data

It is important at this stage to examine key issues in relation to comparative findings within other studies and especially data collected within the period 1993-94. The latter point is especially important in comparing previous study data collected in 1989-1991 with recent data, thus bringing discussions up to date. This section will therefore examine briefly the following:

Comparison of pilot and main study findings;

Comparison with various observational studies;

Cross-validational data;

Interventions and re-measures.

Comparison of pilot and main study findings

The findings of the pilot study (Robinson, 1988, 1990a) are supported by this study. Figure 16 identifies the quantitative similarities between the present study and its pilot.

Data in figure 16 were subject to statistical analysis using Spearman's rank order correlation test to determine the relationship between two data sets, i.e., two wards. The data compared relate to the seven care constructs, i.e., administration/patient supervision; patient functional; patient social; nursing process; miscellaneous; clinical education and domestic categories. Using this routine the following results were obtained: $p<0.025$ one-tailed; $p<0.05$ two-tailed; t-ratio = 4.042; D.F = 5 and rho -.875, thus showing a highly significant relationship.

Such findings offer support for the hypotheses referred to later within this section. Whilst there are still low levels of individualised care, the emphasis placed on this type of care by national health policies during the three years which have elapsed since the pilot has obviously had its effect (see, for example, Department of Health, 1989a, 1992, 1993b). This, together with certain local initiatives (Carton et al, 1990; Robinson, 1990b) may well have contributed to the observed increase in individualised care activity.

Due to the shift in observational criteria and method which has occurred during the last two decades, not all data are transferable for purposes of making useful and valid comparisons. Therefore data will only be presented and discussed where methods and categories are congruent.

Comparison of findings with various observational studies

Comparison with Cormack's data Interesting comparisons have already been highlighted within Figures 6 and 8 of the study findings, and of the shifts occurring between pilot and main study (see Figure 16).

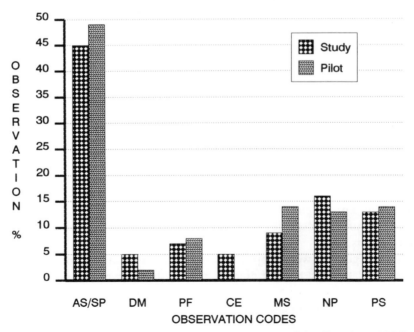

Figure 16 Total ward observations (comparison with pilot data 1988)

Data comparisons were made within the pilot study (Robinson, 1988, 1990a) with data from the work of Cormack (1976), which showed interesting similarities. Figure 17 shows a comparison between Cormack's data and the present study data from R3 ward. Similarities exist in all categories except clinical education and nursing process behaviours (this latter was not introduced at the time).

Data in figure 17 were subjected to statistical analysis using Spearman's rank order correlation test. The data compared relate to the seven care constructs, ie, administration/patient supervision; patient functional; patient social; nursing process; miscellaneous; clinical education and domestic categories. The results were found to be not significant. However, after removing clinical education and nursing process categories the results became significant: $p < 0.025$ one-tailed; $p < 0.05$ two-tailed; t-ratio = 3.576; D.F = 3 and rho = 0.9.

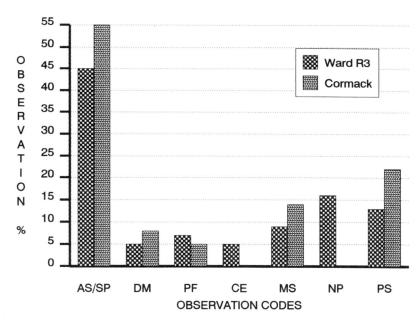

Figure 17 Total ward observations (comparison with Cormack 1976)

These data indicate that, although there is emphasis on individualised care, and clearly this is increasing, little has changed over almost two decades. Data presented earlier also support this proposition (see, for example, Thompson, 1979; Green, 1987; Barrowclough, 1984).

The importance of validating findings by collection of data using two or more methods (triangulation), and especially comparisons made utilising external instruments, is of special importance in verifying findings and validating measures (Denzin, 1970). Prior to collection of observational data within the external location (E1 ward), Psychiatric Audit (Hurst, 1988) had been used in that location (see Annexe K).

The findings using Psychiatric Audit (Owens, 1989) which was completed just prior to data collection in the present study, were adjusted to provide a valid comparison with the results of the present study. Here there was a unique opportunity to compare results obtained by using two different methods of data collection on the same ward within similar time periods and by two separate data collectors. Figure 18 shows the relevant comparisons. As can be seen there are considerable similarities between indirect care and direct/group care to patients. In fact, there is only a three percent difference in the frequencies concerned.

These findings further validate the ward observation schedule and its interpretation. Perhaps more important are the remarkable similarities in the types and amount of care that patients in all observed locations receive. This emphasises the considerable amounts of time not spent with patients which occupy the waking day and appear to waste valuable nursing skills (Cormack, 1983; Street, 1982).

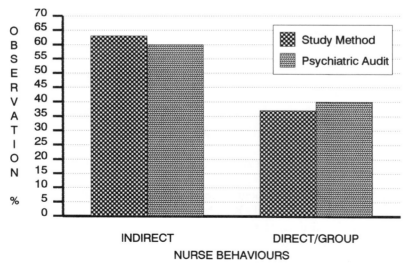

Figure 18 Comparison of study data with psychiatric audit data (E1)

The similarities within the various contexts of psychiatric nursing seem to suggest that nursing activity has changed little over the last decade and is top heavy with administrative and similar non-caring duties (Akinsanya, 1985). These absorb swathes of nursing time and keep skilled staff from dealing with the needs of patients (Cormack, 1983). Similarly, substantial nursing skills (that is, those possessed by ward sisters, charge nurses and staff nurses) are to some degree unused; whilst nursing auxiliaries, who are relatively unskilled, bear the brunt of nursing care. Urgent consideration of current skills deployment is needed to ensure deployment in direct relation to patients' individual needs.

Comparison with general nursing data

Comparisons with data obtained from the general nursing field were also made in order to examine "within" and "between" relationships. Within the hand-held computer programme (Robinson, 1993), which was a computerised version of the observational data collection methods of this study, data were collected within a day surgical ward. Care constructs were validated by general nurses and subsequent modifications made (see Table 26).

Figure 19 highlights emerging trends affecting both the study behaviours and general nursing behaviours. Comparison of indirect and direct group care is made because these care categories can be more accurately compared with external data, and especially with data collected using other methods.

Firstly, Figure 19 overleaf reveals some remarkable similarities within the main study (R3 ward) and a general ward within a Trust Hospital (G1). Supporting evidence for these comparisons can be found in Annexe L. Close similarities exist within the broad context of direct and indirect care types. In other words, almost twice as much time is spent by nurses away from direct contact with patients as in their direct care (see also, for example, Cormack, 1976; Street, 1982; Hurst and Howard, 1988; Robinson, 1990a; Hurst, 1993).

145

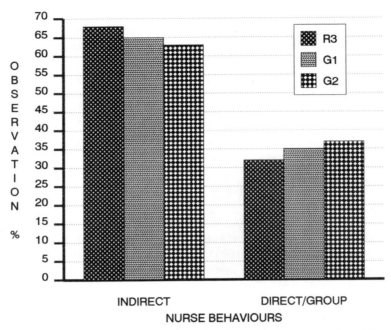

Figure 19 Comparison of nurse behaviours (current study with general nursing)

Qualitative details reveal further similarities in the heavy burden of administrative duties performed by nurses, which account for up to twenty five percent of their time. These absorb the time of skilled nurses, keeping them from much-needed patient care. Similar qualitative details show low frequencies of individualised care, especially within the context of data from the general nursing sample, where it accounted for only six-and-a-half percent of activities. Such low levels of individualised care and other direct care types closely resemble the task-orientated care common a decade and more ago (Hardy and Engel, 1987).

Regarding the G2 category within Figure 19, this reflects data collected by means of a nurse self-recording system. These data were collected by nurses within the same surgical ward during 1992 as part of the Trust Hospital's staffing activity programme (Staffing Activity Analysis, Ward 3A, 1992) (see Annexe M for results).

Close correlations can be found within all three representations (Figure 19) which support broad similarities between aspects of general nursing care and aspects of both mainstream psychiatric and forensic psychiatric nursing care. There is, in fact, only a five percent variance between the three data sets. These data offer further support for two different audit data collection methods finding similar results, (Denzin, 1970); which provides further validation of findings using the ward observation schedule. Clearly these observational instruments display a similar ability to capture broadly congruent patterns of nursing behaviour. The main difference lies in the ability of the ward observation schedule to describe activity in qualitative detail.

In order to extend comparisons and update the exercise, Figure 20 shows data obtained in recent analogous studies (Curl, 1993; Robinson, 1993). These studies display results similar to those of the main study. As part of the trials of clinical data collection using hand-held computers, data were collected from R5 ward (a female mental health ward); R6 ward (an integrated ward for people with learning disabilities); R4 ward (a ward for women suffering from personality disorders); R3 ward (the main study) and G1 ward from the general nursing context. Similar data have been obtained from other wards in Rampton Hospital; and these wards are selected as displaying broadly representative findings since space precludes the presentation of all available data.

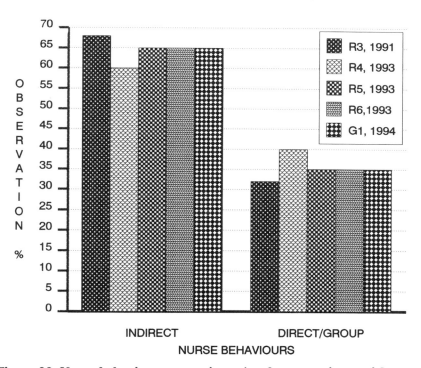

Figure 20 Nurse behaviour comparisons (study comparisons with recent data)

These data show remarkable similarities with those presented earlier. Again we see relatively low levels of direct patient care; and up to twice as much time spent in indirect care (Cormack, 1976; Street, 1982; Hurst and Howard, 1988; Robinson, 1990a; Hurst, 1993). There is only an eight percent variance between the study data collected in 1991 and recent data collected in 1993 and 1994. Supporting data can be found within Annexes N to P.

In support of these comparisons, it is noted that Rhys-Hearn (1979a) found data concerning nursing activities obtained in one ward compared closely with data obtained in other units, despite structural and process differences between the various settings. These findings indicate some potentially important trends within the delivery of nursing care; and there are implications for the close examination of clinical, management and educational issues in relation to change. However, some might argue that the similarities may be artifacts resulting from inflexibility of the research instruments used.

Interventions and re-measures

Pursuing the hypothesis that, following planned intervention, there would be a significant increase in direct care interactions, opportunities arose to collect data, carry out relevant interventions, and re-measure. This had the additional effect of augmenting the original study data with further relevant data recently collected. Within the hand-held computer trials (Robinson, 1993), which use an electronic version of the ward observation schedule, data were collected on two wards.

First, as part of the introduction of a Snoezelen facility, nurses on R6 ward asked if they could have a baseline measure of nursing activity. This, it was posited, would enable them to redirect resources and plan individual care for patients more effectively. Data collection was carried out in June, 1993; and the relevant part of the feedback (that is, direct and indirect care types) appears in Annexe O. Following the installation of the Snoezelen facility, associated with planned individual care programmes, a re-measure took place in December, 1993 (also see Annexe O) to determine what impact these had had on nurse-patient activities.

As can be seen from Figure 21, there has been an increase in direct activity involving patients of four percent. This resulted from the involvement of staff participating within care programmes with patients within the Snoezelen facility. Whilst the Snoezelen programme has yet to be evaluated systematically in terms of patient outcomes, anecdotally the quality and delivery of care seem considerably improved; with informal accounts stressing decreased maladaptive behaviours and an undeniable significant increase in the frequency of nurse-patient interactions.

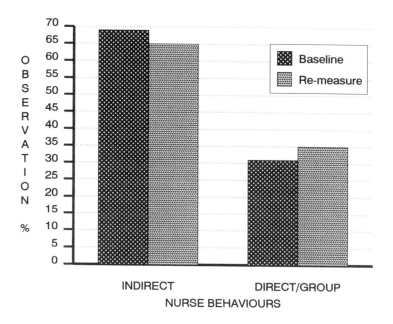

Figure 21 **Comparison of baseline data following intervention and remeasure**

Regarding flexibility of the instrument, such measurable shifts in behavioural frequencies serve as additional evidence. Equally important is the fact that, given re-educative strategies, appropriate support and innovative patient programmes, changes can be brought about which can significantly improve both the quality of health care delivered by nurses and the quality of life experienced by patients (Ashworth, 1985; Green, 1987; Donabedian, 1993).

Secondly, as part of female personality disorder unit research evaluation, baseline measures of nurse-patient activities were obtained in 1992 (see Annexe P). Following this recommendations were made to improve individualised care through a clinically based teaching package (Carton, 1990). Unfortunately few of the recommendations were carried out due to adverse effects of patient and staff turnover; but the re-measure was carried out one year later, in January, 1994 (also see Annexe P).

Despite little if any subsequent work being carried out on individual care planning, the comparisons in Figure 22 show a significant increase in frequency of nurse-patient activities. From this it might be inferred that nurses have had considerable input in improving *individual* care to patients because of the increase in *direct* care. However this is not the case. Here it is necessary to point out the advantage of being able to retrieve qualitative detail through precisely described "time capsules" of care, as discussed earlier in this report. Merely quantitative results can sometimes be misleading! Only with the help of precise, descriptive observational details can quantitative measures be truly interpreted (Leininger, 1992).

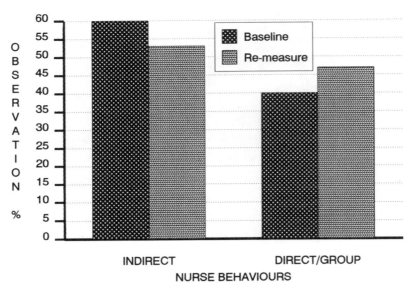

Figure 22 Comparison of baseline data following intervention and re-measure (female personality disorders unit)

In fact, such qualitative details showed that the apparent increase in direct care was due to four patients requiring high levels of one-to-one observation, due to their recent violent and disturbed behaviour. Such observations did not, in fact, form part of planned, *individualised* care. In effect such genuinely individualised care accounted for less than five per cent of activities -far less than the frequencies recorded in other locations and analogous studies; and essentially similar to those obtained in the original baseline measures.

This evidence, whilst reflecting flexibility of the instrument in recording behavioural changes, reinforces the close relationship existing between qualitative and quantitative methods. Without availability of *qualitative* detail, these important issues would go undetected; and it would appear that frequencies of individualised care had increased.

How do we know how much of a particular activity should occur? Whilst this question is partly answered within the qualitative content, through careful examination and clinical decision-making, part must rest on the availability of knowledge. There are considerable valid data available through audits such as that presented in Figure 18. Unfortunately these findings are difficult to track down as they are rarely published. If this type of data were communicated and disseminated, its critical appraisal could contribute more effectively to a body of knowledge that may be used to determine national or local levels of care, and the relevant cultural comparisons needing to be made (Kleinman, 1987).

Recent data from two extensive studies of nursing activity (Department of Health, 1988; Hurst, 1992) show that nurses spend between thirty five percent and forty-five percent of their time giving direct patient care. Data differ from site to site; and Hurst points out some underlying reasons for these differentiae, including development in ward management; employment of ward clerks; ward-based nurse education assessments; and the increasingly technical nature of nursing.

Whilst the latter is more prominent within general nursing, the other issues are certainly relevant within internal contexts. Regarding the levels of direct care types, these are unequivocally supported by the findings of the present study. This provides further evidence for the proposition that the general pattern of nursing activity at Rampton Hospital is not too dissimilar from that occurring in other nursing contexts.

Recent studies also appear to show that levels of direct care are falling (Hilton, 1988; Hurst, 1992; Hurst and Quinn, 1992). So far, this does not appear to be the case within Rampton Hospital. Figure 20 shows an increase in direct care of eight percent between 1991 and 1993.

Indicators have emerged within the present study regarding anticipated ranges of behaviours such as those associated with individualised care: and with their help it is possible to form an empirical judgement regarding performance levels in order to raise standards of care. However this approach will not in itself ensure *quality* rather than *quantity*. Hurst (1993) points out that it is not easy to demonstrate the relationship between frequency of nursing activity (quantity) and associated quality of performance.

It is not surprising that this problem exists, given the quantitative nature of many "quality instruments". Qualitative detail highlighting deficits is crucial here, as is demonstrated within the present study. If it is to become possible to examine care and alter and manipulate it, then precise research-based details are required concerning the processes of care (Aggleton and Chalmers, 1986). Such detailed descriptive accounts start to give insights into the nature of interactions and behaviours, permitting more valid judgements to be made regarding their "quality".

Almost all the nurses within the internal and external locations felt that they had little support with introduction of the nursing process. Most felt that they had to "get on with it" at the time; a finding which is well documented by the low achieved frequencies of individual care for patients.

Whilst feeling relatively unprepared, almost all nurses felt that care planning throughout the introduction of the nursing process had particular advantages (Kitson, 1986). Being more involved, being more able to meet patients' needs, and achievement of greater consistency of care were felt to be important advances in nursing care delivery. However, in one external location (E1 ward) nurse informants felt that there were no major advantages; but did recognise it as a tool to help people "think more logically". Whilst it was felt that advantages outweighed disadvantages, the latter reflected popular beliefs regarding the heavy resultant burden of paperwork and its effect in reducing valuable nursing time which could be spent with patients.

The deficits in educational opportunities for nurses to gain appropriate skills in care planning are reflected within their ability to describe the four phases of the nursing process. Not all nurse informants in every location were able to describe the four phases: and many missed out one or more of the key stages. In general terms, nurse informants from within Rampton Hospital appeared to have more understanding than those from the external locations: not a surprising result given the considerable (though possibly sometimes misguided) investment of education resources in implementing the nursing process at Rampton Hospital.

The task of defining the nursing process concept presented a similar pattern to that of defining the four stages. Nurse informants were largely able to offer meaningful accounts at various levels of understanding. However, some clearly had little if any understanding of its real nature and intention. Again, some external nurse informants - albeit a minority - admitted to being unable to define its principles.

Whilst most nurse informants were able to give accounts of the practical outcomes of care planning and how it affected patient care, some external nurse informants were unable to do so. Although the majority clearly recognised its benefits, these benefits were seldom translated into empirical components of care reflected within the study. Low empirical levels of care planning activity, despite nurses' recognition of its potential advantages, underline a lack of understanding of operational features of individualised care programmes.

The majority of nurse informants felt that care planning could have a substantial effect on care delivery; but much remains to be done. Not all care staff are yet convinced of the value of the approach; and appropriate education is required. Ideally, such education should be delivered in the workplace, thus minimising theory-practice "blocking" which has been a problematic issue in the past.

These issues were well reflected in nurse informants' views about the need to monitor the nursing process. Such monitoring would enable and help justify more support; resulting in increased learning opportunities. Education requires effective delivery at "grass roots" level. Similarly, managers need to support nursing staff by freeing-up resources enabling nurses to respond to patient needs through the use of systematic care planning.

Patients' perceptions of care planning

The concept of patients' involvement as consumers of care breaks away from maternalistic traditional nursing in health care. Involvement of patients in planning their own care now means that they are more likely to feel involved. The nursing process model represents a significant step towards patient involvement in care planning, provided it is systematically and effectively used. However, whilst care provision has moved considerably forward much remains to be done.

Most patient informants felt that there was always a nurse available if they required someone to talk to. Whilst many spoke about the key nurse, some informants felt that, because nurses were assigned to them, resultant relationships were somewhat artificial. In addition, an interesting point was that some patients felt socially restricted because of the key nurse system.

Such patients felt restricted by being assigned to a key nurse; and did not wish to be confined to one nurse in this way. Rather, they wished to develop relationships with whoever they felt able to, or shared specific interests with. These issues begin to challenge the key nurse concept, even if the challenge is restricted to giving more thought and understanding to the flexibility of patients' relationships with nursing staff.

Communication is an essential part of care planning, with the patient being the notional focal point. Patients felt that, whilst there were always nursing staff to talk to, access was sometimes dependent on how busy they were with other duties. Similarly, patients felt that information had to be asked for repeatedly. Observational data reflect relatively infrequent nurse-initiated interactions, as well as high proportions of staff time spent in administrative (ward office) duties. There is clearly a need for reappraisal of staff workloads in favour of opportunities for communicative and interactive work with patients.

Despite these issues, patient informants felt that they were involved in discussions about their care. Quite remarkably, some patients could describe their care plans in considerable detail. Taken together with the foregoing, these findings suggest that, whilst nurses involve patients in routine communication such as care planning, little seems to happen in the social contexts outside of these situations. Similarly, involvement of patients in care planning appears to be somewhat ad hoc. These impressions were supported by ward-based observations, where interactions tended to be patient-initiated more frequently than nurse-initiated.

The above findings indicate that nurse-patient relationships, and especially therapeutic strategies for helping patients gain confidence, require significant development. Similarly, the assignment of key nurses to patients seems to restrict communication and development of other relationships. Whilst this is certainly not the intent, the role of the key nurse appears an extremely important issue in determining the character and quality of relationships between patients and nurses.

Although some patients were able to describe their care plans, they had mixed feelings regarding interventions related to them. Some patients felt that they were receiving appropriate care on a regular basis; but others could not relate to how nurses were attempting to help them. If the low observed levels of care planning and individualised care are considered here, then it is not surprising that patients cannot remember direct care inputs.

Ad hoc interventions and care planning ostensibly not linked to patient need serve to reinforce such dissatisfactions. Patients were frequently unable to trace the "critical link" between current rehabilitation therapies and the reason(s) for their initial admission. Once more in this connection, low frequencies of nurse-patient communication need close examination in relation to establishing more therapeutic relationships with patients.

Multidisciplinary involvement in care planning

Given the sporadic involvement of patients in care planning; the generally low levels of individualised care; documentary deficits; and clear lack of relevant education, it might be assumed that multidisciplinary support would not exist. By contrast, psychologists, educationists and members of other care disciplines are keen to become involved. Current related moves towards collaborative efforts on behalf of patients are well recognised within the present study; and provide a positive move towards genuinely therapeutic care.

Within the current climate of rapid change, the potential advantages of multidisciplinary care are not appreciated by all clinicians. Thus some nurses feel under threat that substantial elements of their role set may be "taken away" by members of other care professions. Apprehension regarding such "role erosion" was obvious in the comments of nurse informants in the present study.

Nonetheless, most nurse informants felt that multidisciplinary professionals should be involved in individual care planning. Different views, it was felt, would provide information about specific patients that may otherwise be unavailable. This information could act as a major resource for nurses. Paradoxically, although nurses spoke about carers being involved, few care plans existed where true multidisciplinary working took place. As nurse informants recognised, valuable information and workload contributions in shared care planning were being lost.

The notion that nursing care plans "belonged" to nurses was a major issue for nurse informants, who frequently spoke proprietarily of multidisciplinary involvement only "if appropriate". Clearly, these nurses felt threatened by what they perceived as a "takeover" or "invasion" of their role. The locus of control for multidisciplinary involvement should remain firmly with the nurses. A minority of two nurse informants felt that other disciplines should become appreciably more involved, especially in "hands-on" care of patients.

From these data it would appear that support for other disciplines' involvement in care planning is clearly evident; but many negative attitudes require to be overcome. Nurses still feel threatened by non-nursing staff interventions; and remain protective of their territory. Much can be gained by exercises in collaborative care planning and delivery, involving multidisciplinary clinical teams. Part of the problem may well lie in the ad hoc initiation of nursing process, during which scant attention was paid to philosophies of collaborative care; with subsequent lack of appropriate educational dialogue and necessary support.

Future education and training programmes clearly need to promote and involve members of related disciplines; ensuring that the patient becomes (or remains) the focal point of shared care planning activities.

Testing study hypotheses

Measurability of nursing care behaviours

The application of relatively insensitive quantitative measures has led to a more or less static design in quality studies (Field and Morse, 1985). The present study has shown that deficits recognised within the literature can be modified in order to elicit new knowledge, regarding both the evolution of methods, and the empirical nature of forensic psychiatric nursing care. The aim throughout has not been to seek to undermine other studies; but rather to build on their important and often pioneering work.

In order to pursue the measurability of nursing behaviours, this study is indebted to the contributions of authors such as Hurst and Howard, 1988;

Goldstone, 1987; Wandelt and Ager, 1978; Phaneuf, 1976; Brooking, 1986; King et al, 1971; Reed, 1978; Moores and Moult, 1979; Mulligan, 1973; and Rhys-Hearne, 1977, for their considerable work in developing observation methods.

Using Leininger's (1986) conceptual theory-generating model, it has been possible to develop care constructs appropriate to psychiatric and to forensic psychiatric nursing (see Tables 23 to 26). The ward observation schedule, building upon descriptive recording methods initiated by King et al, 1971, and Reed, 1978, has made it possible to record precise details of care processes in descriptive form. Subsequent electronic data recall through string-scanning searches has enabled not only quantitative, categorical analysis; but also detailed descriptive accounts of care. Therefore the hypothesis *"that both mainstream psychiatric nursing and forensic psychiatric nursing may be seen as sub-sets of a nursing culture..."* has been well supported within this study. Similarly, it has shown that describing care from the actors' point of view (Field and Morse, 1985; Leininger, 1975) is particularly useful when little is known about a nursing culture. In this case the culture under study has been that of forensic psychiatric nursing care. Using Leininger's theory-generating model (Leininger, 1986) it was possible to develop quantitative categorisations of care (care constructs) through descriptive accounts of care processes. Therefore the hypothesis *"that it is possible to combine both qualitative and quantitative methods to reflect the characteristics of nursing care..."* has also been upheld by the findings of the study.

Similarities between mainstream and forensic psychiatric nursing care

Similarities between mainstream and forensic psychiatric nursing care have been discussed earlier in relation to quantitative measures; and close relationships established. These are highlighted within Figures 6 and 8, where there are remarkably similar patterns emergent in the eight broad categories of nursing care: that is, administrative activities; patient supervision; patient social care; nursing process related activities; and miscellaneous behaviours. Further similarities will now be identified and described in qualitative terms.

Within the care constructs, data reveal that "mainstream" forensic psychiatric nursing care is not too dissimilar from the forensic version offered at Rampton Hospital. Prima facie, it might therefore be assumed that the only difference between psychiatric and forensic psychiatric nursing care contexts would be the security factors. This was certainly the case at Rampton Hospital, where supervision of patients was closely linked to perceptions of their "dangerousness". Conversely, within external locations supervisory behaviours were more assessment-oriented.

156

In all locations, during activities relating to patient supervision, there was a scenario in which nurses were often just "around" should something untoward happen. This "trouble-shooting" mode was especially evident when, on occasions, patients sought attention several times before interventions took place. This degree of imperviousness to non-disruptive attention-seeking was again reinforced by low observed levels of direct care; and an accompanying lack of planned intervention that would involve targeted therapeutic outcomes.

All locations (including the general hospital location) saw considerable staff time spent in ward offices carrying out clerical duties (see also Street, 1982). The "tying up" of senior qualified nurses, professionally skilled staff, in mundane administrative roles is a problem recognised for more than two decades (see, for example, Cormack, 1976, 1983). In the case of recent data obtained from the general nursing context, despite the involvement of a ward clerk, nurses were still swamped by clerical duties.

Whilst forming an important part of ward routine, such activities need careful consideration with regard to possible redirection of professional skills. Similarly, re-education and provision of appropriate support in condensing paperwork, together with its effective use, is long overdue. Until these issues are tackled, patients will continue to get the smaller fraction of available nursing time.

"Overcaring" for patients was a consistent feature within all locations. Often patients received inappropriate care; which may have been due to a lack of, or poor, patient assessment. If patients are to benefit maximally from therapeutic inputs, then these must be carefully structured in relation to their needs. Doing things for them which they can clearly do for themselves is of little value. A specific example of "overcaring" was in relation to domestic chores, where nurses constantly fetched and carried for able-bodied patients.

By contrast, patients must be assisted with their priority needs if their health status and achievements are to be enhanced. Effective care planning is the logical vehicle here, with special reference to assessment: but clearly much work needs to be done for this to become effective.

Regarding education, consistent within all locations was a lack of relevant tutorial input; also a not uncommon finding in Cormack's (1976) data. Responsibility for education in matters relating to nursing process seemed to rest with ward team members, who often had little time available for the task. Whilst all clinicians should be involved in clinically-based education, this should not be at the expense of low levels of direct patient care.

The considerable amount of student nurses' time spent in preparation for various educational tests appeared to leave them little time for involvement in interactive care. Tutors rarely found time to support student nurses on the wards; a factor which tended to result in much of their "educational" time being spent away from patients, instead of participating in guided patient care (see also Davis, 1983).

With the contemporary emphasis on individual care and patient needs, there is a case for student nurses to undertake more practical involvement with patients. This situation appeared widespread in the various locations under study; and is one critical finding among the considerable number which tend to support the hypothesis *that there are marked similarities in the pattern of operational care behaviours* throughout the study locations.

Differences between mainstream and forensic psychiatric nursing care

The major difference between observed "mainstream" and forensic psychiatric nursing care appeared to occur in relation to "supervision" of patients. Whilst frequencies were similar in both cases, qualitative profiles of such supervision were somewhat different.

The potential dangerousness of Rampton Hospital patients meant that considerable time was spent in preventive supervision of patients, thus supposedly ensuring that no harm came to other patients or to nursing staff. Overtly preventive supervision of this type was not encountered to the same extent in the external observational locations.

Social interactions differed in frequency. Generally there appeared to be less social chat with patients in external locations; in one of which nurse-patient communication appeared rare. "Socialising" tended to be patient-initiated rather than staff-initiated, indicating a somewhat one-sided relationship. Cormack also observed this phenomenon as far back as 1976. Effective communication and resultant therapeutic relationships between patients and nurses may be considered crucial to the care process; and considerable efforts to nurture these are still clearly required.

Nurses in the Rampton Hospital wards tended to be "overcaring" in comparison with their peers in external locations. Whilst this was perhaps to be expected on R1 ward, due to the severe learning disabilities of its female residents, surprisingly it was also noticeable on the rehabilitation ward (R2).

By contrast, external wards reflected a more "encouraging" approach to care, in which patients were allowed to do more for themselves. It should, however, be borne in mind that the "security factor" within the Rampton context tended to contribute to the greater frequency of "overcaring" behaviours observed.

Here the strict security procedures (for example, the locking away of all cutlery at times other than mealtimes) meant that even the setting of tables was done for patients. Such tasks are, of course, part of everyday living in the external world; and taking them away tends to increase institutionalisation and to depersonalise patients (Kitson, 1986; Thompson, 1979).

There is obviously a need to explore this "security-therapy" paradox, which otherwise will continue to vitiate rehabilitative care; and to search for model situations to encourage initiative and individuality, whilst not putting other patients or nurses unnecessarily at risk.

Nursing process behaviours were significantly greater in frequency within internal locations than in external wards. However, low levels of direct care were recorded in all locations; and these need to be increased in the Rampton context as elsewhere. The initial input from specially-appointed nursing process coordinators within Rampton Hospital had clearly helped to "routinise" the process to a greater extent than was the case in the external locations.

However, external locations appeared to be better geared to the admission needs of the patients. Such variation gives rise to the considerable work remaining to be undertaken in education of nursing staff in planning and delivery of individualised care. Relative frequencies of nursing process-related activities was one of the areas in which it was possible clearly to demonstrate *"that there are significant differences observable between internal and external contexts"*.

Relationship of care documentation to care delivery

Few studies have reported the relation of documented care to empirical components (Hayward, 1986). This study sought further to clarify the relationship by comparing care plans (by means of the documentary analytic checklist) with ward-based observations (by means of the ward observation schedule).

Documentary evidence, whilst showing various deficits, contained at the very least details of care that was expected to be given. The observational data left no doubt that empirical care in all locations reflected planned care; although there were considered to be low levels of nurse-patient interaction. In addition, many such interactions were based upon patient-initiated behaviours rather than on nurse-initiated therapies or social interventions.

This uncoordinated approach seemed to reflect uncertainty as to timely and appropriate use of care planning strategies. The aim of nursing education effectively to prepare nurses for an approach to individualised care (Davis, 1986b) needs vigorously addressing within each of the study contexts. The current, relatively unsystematic approach, together with evidence of excessively generalised and unfocused care planning notes, reflected the previously reported lack of training and skills within care planning in the wider nursing context (see, for example, Sheehan, 1982, 1986, 1989).

In relation to patient need, care plans written within Rampton Hospital tended to reflect issues relating to activities of daily living, rather than attempting to address possibly less obvious and deeper problems, such as social skills deficits relating to index offenses and reasons for admission. This is clearly a situation that requires addressing, given the current climate of patient need. In general terms the hypothesis *"that documented care reflects that which is actually given"* is supported with some minor reservations. There was no doubt of the positive relationship between planned care and observed care: but planning and progress notes were often too broadly-written to describe operational characteristics of the related empirical care.

Individualised and task-allocated nursing care

Much of the discussion so far has centred upon issues related to individualised care; and it is not the intention to repeat here what has already been said. Individualised care accounted for between twelve and twenty per cent of nursing time across all locations. Similarly, individual care accounted for between twenty-two and twenty-seven percent of nursing activity.

These figures highlight the generally low levels of care planning and direct contact with patients which were observed in all locations (see Figures 6 and 8). Past evidence shows that nurses have tended to care more for an hypothetical "normative" patient rather than for actual individuals (Davis, 1981). Regarding task-allocated care, it is difficult to determine the true extent of such care. Clearly there has been a move away from task-allocated to individualised care; but this presents operational problems, since nurses at times seem unsure what to do next; and often only react to repeated patient initiatives.

The differential frequencies between planned direct care and observed direct care (that is, seven to ten percent of nursing activities) may reasonably be assumed to represent task-allocated care. Additionally, the relatively large amounts of indirect care - for example, care planning; assessment; evaluation; logistics of patient social activities; and related administration - represent considerable frequencies of task-allocated care. Therefore the hypothesis *"that individualised care will occur with less frequency than task-allocated types of care"* was supported. However, task-allocation occurred less frequently in relation to direct care and group care activities. Similarly, the final hypothesis *"that indirect care will account for the largest proportion of nursing activity"* has been shown to be correct for this study.

Nursing process - or multidisciplinary care process?

This study has given accounts of the introduction and contemporary status of the nursing process which are well supported in the literature. For example, Leddy and Pepper (1993) found that, in the reality of contemporary nursing practice, many nurses do not use the nursing process as a deliberate clinical method. This is not surprising in situations where there is sometimes a disturbing lack of related clinical education for nursing staff; and a lack of practical, related experiential opportunities accorded to students.

At its inception, nursing process appeared to offer nurses a systematic approach to the delivery of care; and a chance to take care to the individual (White, 1993). In addition, it was held that the patient would no longer be seen as playing a passive role in his/her care; but would be seen as being centrally involved in related decision-making. Similarly, the concept was seen as developmental, in helping to facilitate the move towards a genuinely research-based profession.

In reality, the notion of achieving individualised care through the nursing process appears to be little advanced, despite a decade-and-a-half of implementation. Even in North America, the founding culture of nursing process, it now appears that there is little evidence of its effective implementation. For example, in a visit to American hospitals, Kirwin (1980) found no evidence that the nursing process as described was practised; and found that the majority of practising nurses had abandoned it as a dream conjured up by educationists, who were thought to be out of touch with the realities of clinical practice.

More recently in Canada, Shea (1986) reported that the number of patients with operational care plans was almost nil. In the case of those patients for whom such care plans had been prepared, most of these were either out of date or had been abandoned. More recently still, Lawler (1991) describes the nursing process as a "relative failure".

The debate finds little fault with the underlying aspirations of the advocates of nursing process towards genuinely individualised care; but rather with the sometimes socially and educationally inept manner in which attempts were made to introduce it; and with the lack of systematic organisational and educational support which it obviously requires if it is to succeed.

Dukes and Stewart (1993) note that it is perhaps not the concept of nursing process itself, but rather its *lack of implementation*, with which nurses have not yet come to terms. One of the fundamental issues seems to be that the nursing process has not been seen to be derived from clinical practice. Quite clearly, both nurses and members of other care disciplines need to own the approach, and be centrally involved in it, if it is to succeed to any degree.

Unfortunately the term nursing process appears to have encouraged some members of the nursing profession to take a proprietorial approach, which has rarely involved members of other disciplines. In this respect the term nursing process now seems somewhat dated; and therefore does little to enhance perceptions of the nursing contribution to health care.

By contrast, contemporary approaches to health care stress multidisciplinary involvement, where by consensus the products of shared assessment, care planning, implementation and evaluation can be brought together successfully, to the satisfaction both of the patient and of all members of the care team.

Towards a multidisciplinary care process

The notion of individualised care programmes should not be lost; but the nursing process label needs to be reconsidered. Since the nursing process as currently practised has never succeeded in bridging the theory-practice gap, careful consideration of its status is needed; together with strategic discussions on how best to take forward related initiatives on individualised care.

To be fair, the analysis must take account of the impacts of current organisational issues. Rapid changes in the health care system appear to have placed some constraints on the care nurses can give; partial results of which may be increasingly high levels of administrative work, and correspondingly lower levels of direct care. Of potentially even greater significance to psychiatric patients are the frequency and quality of interpersonal interactions which they find it possible to achieve with nurses (Peplau, 1994). In this respect, nurses, in collaboration with other mental health professionals, need to take a step back and re-examine some fundamental issues of practical care delivery.

Education and clinical practice managers now need to bring about substantial change towards, as well as promoting investment in, *multidisciplinary* individualised care. If the patient's needs are to be seen as central to care, and patients are to be seen as equal partners in making related care decisions, then individualised care programmes represent a key area, not simply in nursing, but in *multidisciplinary* care research.

Careful debate now needs to take place, to ensure that valuable elements of current investment are not lost; that nurses and other care workers have the requisite opportunities to practice important care planning skills; that due attention is given to overcoming the theory-practice gap; and that relevant education is itself based on substantive research activities, preferably conducted in an ethos of inter-professional collaboration.

Implications for community-based care

A major ostensive function of hospitalisation is to help patients resolve their problems, thus enabling them to return to their communities in the shortest possible time. It is the nurse's responsibility, working both with the patient and with other professionals, to move towards this aim.

Here individualised care planning can have an important part to play. A recent study has identified shortfalls in patient preparation for community care and emphasised the importance of care planning based upon individual needs (Reed and Robinson, 1993). Within this study patients discharged into a range of community settings frequently spoke about deficits, such as life and living skills - in many cases lost through institutionalisation - in their preparation for discharge.

By means of rigorous assessment and effective recording, using systematic approaches to care delivery identical with, or akin to, the nursing process, care inputs can be planned, implemented and monitored. These can have considerable benefits in planning community resettlement of patients; as well as in indicating levels of achievement in terms of outcomes for the personal benefit of the patient.

Much emphasis is currently being placed on such outcomes as possible indicators of patients' progress and of the quality of the care given. If such systematic approaches are implemented more effectively in the practice context, with agreed levels of patient-nurse interaction, then indicators of quality and patient outcomes will develop organically out of the care process, given that such developments are carefully and systematically monitored.

Finally, the recent review of mental health nursing (Butterworth, 1994) raises some interesting and exciting challenges. Most important in relation to this study is its ninth recommendation: *"that mental health nursing should be arranged to ensure that nurses spend the majority of their time responding to the needs of people who use services"*. Empirical levels of direct care, and especially of individualised care, remain to be established in the wider context. Similarly, there are as yet no *formal* guidelines as to how much individual care patients should receive. The Butterworth review challenges nurses by *informally* indicating a desirable level as comprising "the majority" of their time.

If direct patient care is to benefit from "the majority" of available nursing time, then potentially effective care delivery systems, such as that outlined more than two decades ago in the nursing process, need urgent reappraisal in terms of what they have yet to offer to a contemporary, multidisciplinary ethos of community-based psychiatric care.

Contributions to new knowledge

Related theoretical propositions

The study data have been shown to support the hypotheses, most of which are recurring themes throughout the investigation. Such hypothetical propositions relating to the empirical nature of forensic psychiatric nursing may be considered to be contributions to new knowledge since confirmatory studies had not been carried out previously within the context of the three English special hospitals. Theoretical propositions emergent within the study include the following:

that both mainstream psychiatric nursing and forensic psychiatric nursing may be seen as sub-sets of a nursing culture;

that it is possible to combine both qualitative and quantitative descriptors to reflect the characteristics of nursing care;

that there are marked similarities between locations in the patterns of operational care behaviours;

that there are significant differences observable between internal and external contexts;

that documented care reflects that which is actually given;

that individualised types of nursing care will occur less frequently than task-allocated types of nursing care;

that indirect care will account for the largest proportion of nursing activity.

In addition to knowledge generated from hypotheses it has been possible to generate from the study data the following empirical propositions:

that there is a theory-practice gap resulting from little or inappropriate tutorial input at ward level;

that the low frequencies of staff-initiated interactions reflect a general "social distance" in staff-patient relationships;

that the dearth of individualised care observed still reflects care patterns described almost two decades ago;

that the frequency of individualised care is increasing in the Special Hospital context under study;

that direct nursing care is restricted because of the overburden of administrative duties;

that there are broad similarities in overall behavioural patterns of nursing staff, whether observed within forensic psychiatric nursing; "mainstream" psychiatric nursing; or in learning disabilities and general nursing contexts;

that there are broadly similar patterns of administrative behaviour displayed by nursing staff within forensic psychiatric nursing contexts; "mainstream" psychiatric nursing contexts; and in learning disabilities and general nursing contexts;

that quantitative results can be misleading without the support of qualitative-descriptive evidence;

that it is possible to measure shifts in nursing behaviours following baseline measures in response to appropriate change strategies;

that there is a lack of communication and related relationships between patients and staff;

that there is a dearth of planned therapeutic interventions, relating inter alia to a lack of staff-initiated interactions;

that there is little use of therapeutic nursing skills in relation to individual patient needs;

that there is considerable "overcaring" for patients, especially in the Rampton contexts;

that there is a tendency for security needs to predominate, rather than interventions therapeutically based upon individual needs.

Additionally, the study has helped clarify some important issues highlighted within the pilot study (Robinson, 1988). Firstly, the study has shown that it is possible to describe the nature of nursing care observationally in terms of nursing process and non-nursing process behaviours.

Secondly, it has shown that the clinical characteristics of such nursing care can be analyzed in finer-grained detail than has previously been attempted, without loss of quantitative rigour.

Thirdly, it has shown that, by using combined documentary analytic and observational methods, it is possible to develop reliable comparisons of documented and empirical care.

Finally, it has shown that the instruments used possess generalising properties making them useful in examining wider contexts of nursing care.

Application of anthropological theory

This study has striven to overcome weaknesses noted within the literature through anthropological approaches where its descriptive scientific approach (Leininger, 1992) allows fine-grained description of human behaviours not seen within current quality studies. Such descriptive approaches have allowed the researcher to "live and capture" life experiences of those living and working within the contexts under study (McCaugherty, 1992a). The translation of findings into terms and categories that allow cross-cultural comparisons is considered to be the anthropologist's ultimate, most sophisticated step (Kleinman, 1987).

Anthropology is essentially a field of detailed, intensive single-culture study, in which comparisons are made by a scholarly review of the literature on other cultures (Kleinman and Good, 1985). Similarly, the translation of findings into categories (or, in this case, care constructs) allows cultural and cross-cultural comparisons within and between internal and external locations (Kleinman, 1987).

However, whilst some of the care constructs presented within Leininger's theory-generating model (see Table 23) lend themselves to most health care settings, they are presented at too generalised a level to describe the nature of nursing interventions within forensic and mainstream psychiatric care. Thus each construct reflects a theoretical meta-description rather than reflecting the interpretation of empirical care processes within a ward environment. Similarly, in order to utilise the model effectively, "care" must be understood, represented and fitted into the cultural language of the specific organisation (Kleinman, 1987).

Within the pre-pilot study (Robinson, 1987) fourteen care constructs were identified through detailed observations which are justified through the use of neo-realist theory (Russell, 1912, 1914, 1921). Such theory justifies detailed observation providing it is subject to rigorous inter-rater reliability checks where two persons perceive similar perspectives and offer similar interpretations of events. High levels of inter-rater reliability were subsequently recorded within this study.

Therefore, the "meta-constructs" offered in Leininger's theory-generating model (Leininger, 1986) are reinterpreted as "operational" constructs meaningful within the area under study. The pilot study (Robinson, 1988) identified a further care construct (clinical education) which was not represented in the earlier ward observations. Thus, for the current study, fifteen care constructs were identified. The care constructs which then represented forensic and "mainstream" psychiatric nursing care are as follows:

Table 24 Initial care constructs used in present study

1 administrative-supervisory
2 supervision of patients
3 care assessment (implicit)
4 care assessment (explicit)
5 care planning (implicit)
6 care planning (explicit)
7 care implementation (implicit)
8 care implementation (explicit)
9 care evaluation (implicit)
10 care evaluation explicit
11 patient-social (general)
12 patient-functional (general)
13 clinical education
14 domestic
15 miscellaneous
(each of these care constructs has numerous sub-descriptions within the Ward Observation Schedule)

Detailed ward observations were categorised, but not forced, into the care constructs for quantitative description. A key feature of the observations is the descriptive recording of "time capsules" of care. The technique enables these descriptions to be interrogated at any subsequent period, either for validational purposes or during development of further care constructs.

From inspection of the pilot and pre-pilot data (Robinson, 1987, 1988), similarities began to emerge that enabled hypotheses to be generated and

167

subsequently tested within the present study.

During the later stages of the study, developments outlined elsewhere in this respect have resulted in further analysis and refinement of the care constructs (Robinson, 1993); and these subsequent reformulations are presented in Table 25. They are discussed later when making comparisons with recent data collected in 1993 and 1994 (see Figure 19).

Table 25 Revised care constructs from the current study

1   ward administration
2   patient supervision
3   care planning activity
4   patient social
5   communication with patient
6   communication about patient
7   group therapy
8   medication
9   domestic
10 personal
11 clinical education
12 patient functional
13 off ward duties
14 level of observations
(each of these care constructs has numerous sub-descriptions within the ward observation schedule)

Recent developments from the present study involved electronic data capture, using hand-held computers and a customised electronic report generator, enabling data to be collected within a general nursing context (Robinson, 1993). Subsequently, care constructs were validated for data collection on a day surgical ward within a Trust Hospital. Eight hundred observations were collected, which was within the representative frequency detailed later.

Most existing nursing care constructs were felt to be valid for the new context, with the addition of a "specialist technical procedures" category. Data analysis showed that the care constructs typified care processes very accurately; but required some further, albeit slight, modifications. Therefore the care constructs validated within the general nursing setting are presented in Table 26. From these measurements some inferences can be drawn in terms of comparisons between psychiatric and general contexts of nursing care. (Kleinman, 1987)

Table 26 Care constructs used in the general nursing context

```
 1  ward administration
 2  care planning activity
 3  patient social
 4  communication with patient
 5  communication about patient
 6  medications
 7  domestic
 8  personal
 9  clinical education
10  patient functional
11  off ward duties (with patient)
12  off ward duties (non patient)
13  general procedures
14  special technical procedures
```

Contribution to contextual studies in forensic psychiatric nursing

Whilst considerable research into forensic care issues has been carried out by members of non-nursing disciplines, nursing research is still relatively new to the forensic setting: and few, if any, studies describe the detailed processes of forensic nursing care. Therefore the development of constructs with which to represent forensic nursing care is well justified.

To date, the researcher is not aware of current or past research which attempts to describe in detail the nature and processes of this culture. Recent informal contact with all the English regional secure units, as well as a literature search within the three special hospitals, revealed no studies related to this. The present study has therefore provided a baseline understanding of how nurses interact with patients in such contexts, and the subsequent implications of such interaction, in three distinct ways.

Firstly, it has quantified behaviours and interactions that can be compared in most forensic psychiatric contexts. The validation of these anthropological approaches will allow useful baselines to be set and subsequent re-measures obtained. Such care constructs will allow knowledge to be continually updated and applied to other health care settings for purposes of cross-cultural comparisons (Kleinman, 1987).

Secondly, the study has broken new ground by offering a qualitative approach which is also flexible enough to quantify nursing interactions and behaviours. Equally important is its ability to develop a detailed description of the sub-components of care, which is necessary when studying new social phenomena (Leininger, 1987). The potential richness and retrievability of descriptive data concerning life experiences within this cultural setting are central features of the present study (Akinsanya, 1986; Leininger, 1992). In addition its descriptive approach allows dynamic evolution of care construct representation which accurately mirrors the changing health care context.

Thirdly, through their centrality to the description of care processes, the baseline measures offer important empirical insights as a starting point for change. By remeasurement following implementation of change strategies, cultural and health-related outcomes can be monitored. Although the present study has concentrated almost exclusively on processes of nursing care, such re-measures have important implications for development of future indicators of related outcomes attributable to nursing care.

Contribution to comparative studies in nursing

A number of antecedent observational studies have been carried out into nursing care in various specialities, including mental handicap (Moores and Grant, 1976); psychiatric nursing (Cormack, 1976); acute services (Mulligan, 1972, 1973; Moores and Moult, 1979); and geriatric nursing care (Rhys-Hearne, 1976, 1979). However the nature of such studies is determined:

by their original purposes;

by prevailing concepts of nursing care obtaining at the time of each study;

by rapid social and professional changes occurring since each study;

by disciplinary constraints;

by methodological issues already discussed.

Many previous studies have been concerned with ward staffing to the exclusion of other quality issues; whereas the present study seeks to examine and develop a number of qualitative criteria within forensic nursing care. Similarly, every study is "a child of its time"; concepts of nursing care can, and do, change - and with them the social contexts within which that care is delivered.

For these reasons, some of the excellent formative studies previously mentioned now appear conceptually rather dated; or concerned with issues already solved or no longer professionally to the forefront. However, by far the most important reasons for carrying out the present study relate to disciplinary and methodological shortcomings in the study of contemporary forensic psychiatric nursing care.

There are, quite literally, no systematic empirical studies to date into the nature and quality of psychiatric nursing care, as it is currently being delivered within the Special Hospitals. Under the auspices of the Special Hospital Services Authority, a number of studies are now being set up (of which this is one), with the intention of obtaining valid and reliable empirical data concerning nursing in Ashworth, Broadmoor and Rampton Hospitals.

Without these data, it remains impossible to design and implement a logical, relevant programme of change within the hospitals, considering the critical relation of nursing care to patient progress and ultimate recovery. Similarly, unless such data are forthcoming, no effective baselines can be obtained against which to measure the impacts of any change, either good or bad. This is a situation which cannot continue within a modern forensic nursing service, which must work to therapeutically effective and economically suitable indicators for change.

None of the observational studies of nursing care previously described has dealt with the specific and delicate problems of the forensic psychiatric nursing context; and this is true of contemporary quality studies, as well as the formative methodological studies mentioned above, which were carried out some years ago.

Methodological advances

The present study has seen considerable advances based upon reflection and innovation related to other studies. Ideas have also developed through critical appraisal of this study's methods through dissemination at local and international level (see, for example, Robinson, 1988; 1988a; 1989ab; 1990 acd; 1991ab; 1992a; 1993acdeh; 1994 and 1994a). Such dissemination has ensured critical commentary, advice and support.

Refinement of qualitative indices

A number of observational and quality care studies have contributed invaluably to the groundwork on which this study is based. These include examples of observational audit (eg, Rush-Medicus; QUALPACS; Monitor; Psychiatric Audit); earlier formative observational studies (eg, King, Raynes and Tizard,

1971; Mulligan, 1972, 1973; Moores and Grant, 1978); and documentary audit (eg, Phaneuf, 1976; Hurst, 1987; Brooking, 1988).

A detailed critique of problematic issues relating to the above studies cannot be given here; but a few indications concern disciplinary specificity, quantitative emphasis and smallness of scale (see, for example, Moores and Grant, 1976); limitation of data to acute nursing care contexts; and large-scale quantitative analysis "shaping" the data to the exclusion of qualitative data (see, for example, Moores and Moult, 1979); unsuitability of "activity sampling" as a key to workload in psychiatric nursing contexts (see, for example, Mulligan, 1972, 1973); limitation of data to geriatric nursing care contexts and some pre-study "manipulations" of the observed wards (Rhys-Hearne, 1979).

Similarly, many of these studies were concerned specifically with impacts of staffing on nursing care in unidisciplinary contexts; and not directly with other quality issues. The studies concerned are now some ten to twenty years old; and naturally reflect the rather task-orientated concepts considered appropriate to nursing in the late 1960s and 1970s. None of the observational studies cited (with the exception of Rhys-Hearne in a geriatric care context) tackles the issue of individual care planning, now regarded as a key quality indicator.

The present study strove to build on the important work already carried out within the field of quality studies. Limitations in some of their designs identified by various recent authors made it possible for this study to examine and overcome problematic issues. Doubts about validity and reliability (Smith, 1986; Oliver, 1991) were overcome by systematic inter-rater reliability and validity exercises (Kleinman, 1987). These were also supported by a multi-method approach and by comparison of findings with those of analogous studies using different methods (Denzin, 1970; Cowman, 1993).

Redfern and Norman (1990), stated that most instruments were in need of extensive validity testing in relation to what they purport to measure. this study operationalised Leininger's (1986) theory-generating model to enable development of anthropologically-based care constructs, tending to accurate representation and validity of phenomena under study.

Forcing of complex interactions into inappropriate quantitative measures (Dickson, 1987; Redfern and Norman, 1990) were overcome using a descriptive approach (Leininger, 1992). Describing and recording "time capsules" of care, and coding of qualitative data at the end of observational sessions, allowed careful post hoc consideration to be given to categorisation and moved away from forcing observations into pre-determined categories. In addition, descriptions are not lost as with traditional quantification: hence "time capsules" of empirical care can be recalled at any time from the electronic database.

Balogh (1991) identified current time-sampling techniques and observer interference as problematic. Similarly, these methods failed to capture the true reflection and range of complicated interactions. These problems were overcome in the present study by using thirty-second time-sampling intervals, which made more effective use of observers' time (Robinson, 1988); and started to pick up changing behaviours through a span of four consecutive recordings. Because of the familiarity of the observer to location nursing staff, and the descriptive method of recording, few problems were encountered due to researcher interference with nurses' duties.

These issues are extremely important when considering the measurability of nursing behaviours. Although current quality methods have made important contributions, limitations must still be overcome. Comparisons with data collected by other methods (discussed earlier) must play an important role in validating the current study's ability to measure nursing behaviours.

The researcher has sought to learn from the above issues, and produce a modified method which will avoid some of the pitfalls identified and enrich *qualitative* aspects of the data collected. These studies are seen as formative and vitally important in their own right; and it is not the intention of this study to attempt to discredit them in any way; but rather to build upon their important contributions.

The main innovative features and developments from current quality methods include, firstly a *documentary analytic checklist* designed to assess the care planning records of individual patients. Based on the work of Phaneuf (1976), Hurst (1987) and Brooking (1988), this instrument employs a detailed, fifty-six-item checklist examining in depth each qualitative component of individualised care as outlined within the documentation.

Although the literature offers a steady output of papers examining the theoretical content of each phase of the nursing process, these have seldom been examined as empirical comparisons of care given with care planned (Hayward, 1986). This instrument also includes observational criteria to assess whether care planned and reflected in the documentation is actually carried out.

Secondly, the study utilised a specially designed *ward observation schedule* which examines care processes qualitatively and seeks to avoid categorical "forcing" of observations (see, for example, Barnett and Wainwright, 1987; Redfern and Norman, 1990; Oliver, 1991). Previous observational data sheets examined by the researcher normally seek frequencies of a specific care construct, categorised rather rigidly at a remove from the precise behaviour observed. Thus precise details of the many individual behaviours occurring within such a construct are usually lost. By contrast, instead of ticking categories , the observation schedule allows the researcher to write a brief but careful description of each behaviour observed. This detailed record may then be retrieved at any time during subsequent analysis.

Many previous studies employ a "periodic" time-sampling mode, which unfortunately threatens continuity of observational sequences by concentrating only on what is happening at the end of each three-to-ten minute sequence, thus losing all interim data. Such techniques are both observer-intensive and wasteful, as well as disturbing continuity (Balogh, 1991; Redfern and Norman, 1990). The present study overcame this by employing rotational thirty-second time-sampling, concentrating on one individual for four observations before moving on to the next individual. By this means more detailed and continuous data sequences were obtained.

Finally, the study has shown that quantitative measures can sometimes misrepresent the true picture by giving false indications of shifts in behaviours (see Figure 22). It is therefore important that descriptive accounts verify data shifts and variables influencing these are accounted for. Within this study the descriptive nature of recording, and subsequent analytic retrieval, assist in substantiating such measures and break modest new ground in qualitative methods.

Hurst (1993) indicates that *activity* has not yet established its relationship to *quality*. The methods described above seek to address this issue.

Advances in data capture, analysis and reports

The present study has had many spin-offs, one being the development of electronic data capture and analysis (Robinson, 1993ab; 1994; Curl, Robinson and Reed, 1993). The year-long task of inputting observational data into the database during this study formed the basis for development of related audit software for use with hand-held computers.

The resultant software has already contributed to National Health Service audit programmes; and much interest in the system's potential has been expressed throughout the prison service and in other NHS care contexts.

A further significant innovation relates to retrievability of data and ease, rapidity and flexibility of data-processing. Here the researcher is fortunate in having access to sophisticated modern integrated software for data capture, upload and subsequent analysis, using a hand-held terminal. Software has been customised for the specific purposes of the present study.

Data are entered directly into a computerised data sheet. Not only can nursing behaviours be categorised quantitatively; but also the *repertoire* of behaviours occurring may be specified in verbal detail and in real time. Qualitative aspects of nursing care delivery may be examined and compared within and between wards and internal/external care units by *string-scanning* (word searching) techniques within the resultant electronic database. Here the analysis differs radically from the standard quantitative analyses undertaken in earlier studies, since mainframe computers of the mid-1970s were incapable of sophisticated qualitative data-handling.

Qualitative data-strings are created to form a permanent and readily-accessed record of what actually occurred, minute-by-minute, during observed care sequences. It is hoped that this method may break some new ground within quality studies by making more precise the largely unknown details of various care processes and related behaviours occurring within forensic psychiatric nursing. It is further suggested that they may possess developmental implications for quality audit methods within related care specialities.

Contribution to quality audit

The study has also contributed to quality audit. Observational Standards of Care Audit and Review (OSCAR) (Robinson, 1990b) drew substantially on this study and its pilot (Robinson, 1988). Using the documentary analysis and patient and staff interview data, standard criteria were developed. Fifty-six criteria drawn from the documentary analytic checklist were used; and a further seventy-two patient and staff criteria were derived from responses to interviews. This audit instrument is now in its third draft at Rampton Hospital; is now also in use within Ashworth Hospital; and has recently been accepted as an audit framework for the prison health care service (Harrison, 1994).

The documentary analytic checklist has also become the focus of further research in developing a clinically-based nursing process teaching and learning package (Carton, 1990, 1994). This has seen considerable use within Rampton Hospital; and will shortly be brought to bear on care planning issues in R4 ward.

Related developments in data collection resulted in the Computerised Observational Care Audit (COCA). This project grew through a two-year research project at diploma level (Robinson, 1993; 1993a; Curl et al, 1993); and received two year funding by the Department of Health (£44,000 between 1991 and 1993). Using the ward observation schedule and care constructs developed within the main study, observational audit programmes were developed. The resultant audit is currently in use within Rampton Hospital; and has also been adapted for use in the general nursing field where related audit is currently ongoing.

The development and use of resultant software for hand-held computers has pioneered an innovative method in data collection and analysis. National and international dissemination through conferences is already exerting an influence on the way nursing audit data and observational research data are collected (Robinson, 1993cdefgh).

Derived patient outcome indicators

Whilst the present study has been concerned mainly with the *processes* of care, it has also been possible to identify some indices that may be used in connection with patient *outcome* studies.

Firstly, quantitative measurement of frequency of occurrences of specific care behaviours can form baselines for use as general predictors of nursing performance. Following implementation of appropriate change strategies, remeasures can then be carried out and examined for shifts in frequency of care delivery. As identified in Figure 21, data shifts can be assessed for patient outcomes in relation to changes in practice.

Secondly, qualitative observational details can be examined, compared and contrasted to determine the outcome effects of care delivery. Such qualitative detail not only reinforces quantitative measurement; but also provides precise descriptive details of patient outcomes. It can also be used to monitor longer-term reactions of patients to specific interventions.

Thirdly, documentary analysis of care plans can also be used to identify care delivery specified within the documentation. Deficits, or specifically identified care delivery, can be compared with, and validated against, empirically observed care.

Contribution to new nursing knowledge

The present study has helped clarify the fundamental link between individualised care programmes and quality of care. Because the study is limited to three internal wards at Rampton Hospital and two external wards, it may be considered that little generalisation is possible. However, a growing number of quality-related studies support many of this study's findings; and tend to cross-validate it both for forensic and mainstream psychiatric nursing services. Similarly, both the pilot study (Robinson, 1988) and subsequent recent data derived from the main study yield significantly reliable similarities.

At the very least, within the forensic contexts, the fact that *no* previous systematic, descriptive studies have examined the nature and processes of forensic nursing care makes the current findings within these locations a contribution towards new knowledge. There are also intriguing similarities in quantitative terms with results obtained in other internal wards and external locations.

Relative frequencies of nursing process behaviours are low when compared with other, non-personal aspects of nursing care, such as administrative and supervisory duties. These findings are potentially important in relation to the remarkable similarities existing between internal and external locations in this respect; and especially interesting when compared with observations made in the general nursing context, where, again, important similarities exist.

Whilst there appears to be a steady increase in individualised care programmes in the Rampton contexts, indirect care accounts for more than half of available nursing time. In the contemporary professional climate, which dictates that health care should be based upon individualised assessment, there is still a considerable way to go in reducing this imbalance.

The operational care constructs, which have now held good for over 30,000 observations, have enabled comparisons of different nursing cultures. The remarkable similarities in observed patterns of behaviour between forensic psychiatric nursing care contexts; "mainstream" psychiatric nursing care contexts; and general nursing care contexts, show common themes within nursing. In each case, the considerable time spent away from patients (over fifty per cent of available nursing time) places inevitable resultant stresses on the caring process.

These parallel trends show that, in many ways, forensic psychiatric nursing care is not too dissimilar from that experienced in other psychiatric and general nursing contexts. Whilst activities related to security are more evident within the internal locations, this is often simply a "front" which disguises lack of nursing intervention. What is quite clearly needed here is an adequate frequency of therapeutic interventions which, it is hypothesised, will contribute towards a reduction in "single agenda", security-related activities.

Bridging the theory-practice gap

Theoretical beliefs underlying forensic psychiatric nursing have been based upon traditional values, experience and logic. This study has helped clarify elements of the dichotomy existing between such approaches and contemporary care planning approaches, by describing in detail resultant nursing care.

Theoretical assumptions underlying individualised care, and empirical findings related to them, have been discussed earlier in this report within which contemporary beliefs about deficits in individualised care have been well supported.

Development of appropriate care constructs has allowed the Rampton nursing culture to be studied and comparisons made with external nursing cultures. Use of these care constructs has enabled baseline measures to be taken, and, in some cases, assessed for evidence of change. Subsequent results have facilitated discussion with practitioners to inform practice and advocate employment of suitable change strategies.

Such discussions have enabled clarification of the theoretical beliefs underlying individualised care planning; and their subsequent translation into nursing actions. Remeasures taken subsequent to implementation of change strategies have allowed assessment of the impacts of intervention (see Figure 21); and some bridging of the theory-practice gap through practical application.

Potential benefits to patients and nurses

The first and perhaps most important benefit to patients and nurses is the ability of the latter to receive systematic evidence of the nature of nursing and patient activities. Within cognate studies using hand-held computers, electronic data analysis and next-day feedback of results (Robinson, 1993), nursing staff have been able to use the data in ways previously outlined.

Nursing staff have used the observational data to redirect care processes and make best possible use of scarce nursing resources. Perhaps one of the most important issues relating to this is the rapid feedback of results. This clearly has an advantage for encouraging nurses' perceptions that results are real and relevant. Thus the latency of feedback is appropriate to ensure that patients receive more suitably planned and relevant care.

Similarly the documentary analytic checklist has already yielded benefits for patients and nursing staff. The ward audit developed from this (Robinson, 1990b) has documented more than two hundred subsequent improvements in procedures related to patient care. Consequently the benefits of this study to patients have been appreciable in pointing the way to improvements in the quality of nursing care which they receive.

Carton et al (1990) have developed the documentary analytic checklist to function as a sensitive indicator of specific care planning deficits displayed by individual care planners within a selected nursing care context. Following assessment of deficits, a clinical teaching and learning package is implemented addressing specific deficits in the documentation to enable practice-based learning to take place. This approach to improving acquisition of care planning skills, and subsequent delivery of nursing care, offers considerable potential for reducing the theory-practice gap by demonstrating to clinicians the practical relevance of nursing theory in influencing care delivery in the workplace.

Improvements in care planning skills, and in resultant delivery of individualised care programmes, are among factors responsible for measurable increases in observed frequencies of individualised care behaviours (see Figure 6); with twenty-four per cent of revised nursing activities in this particular unit (R2 ward) now accounted for by nursing process related activities. As a corollary, related staff knowledge and skills, and related standards of patient care, have both appreciably improved.

More general benefits accruing from this study of nursing care will, it is hoped, contribute both to local and to wider contexts of health care. Its methods will allow baseline data to be used by nursing staff, both to understand and to assess their contributions to patient care. Similarly, illustrating the use of such baselines and remeasures will assist in evaluating the quality of service given to patients; and thus hopefully contribute to its gradual improvement.

Additionally, data derived from extended studies of this type will provide information to facilitate resourcing decisions regarding clinical nursing care. These, in turn, will assist in assessing quality care implications; and increase the probability that patients, as consumers, are recipients of consistent, high quality nursing care.

A brief summary of related potential benefits could include the following:

Facilitating nursing evaluations of strengths and weaknesses in existing nursing care;

extending nurses' existing knowledge of differing care delivery systems;

helping nurse educators to utilise knowledge gained to provide current research-based information within basic, continuing and higher education programmes.

Limitations of the study

Most methods for collecting information that attempt to fathom and describe the nature of a culture not previously described frequently elicit more information than was intended (Davis, 1986a). This was certainly the case with observational data in the current study. With hindsight, it may have been less wasteful if observational samples had been slightly fewer.

Whilst the arguments for employing observers familiar with their own wards for purposes of observational data collection were accepted in principle, commitment from some managers was marginal. At one stage it was thought unlikely that observations in one internal location (R1 ward) would ever get under way. Nurses observing in their own wards, even though supernumerary to ward staffing, had to contend with constant interruptions from their "own" patients. Similarly, managers often tried to use them to fill contingent gaps in staffing requirements. These issues took up considerable researcher time in carrying out the necessary re-negotiations.

Although invaluable to the study, the selected external care locations were both at a considerable distance from the researcher's base at Rampton Hospital. Whilst frequent visits for observer support and inter-rater reliability checks were fully met, frequent travelling problems were encountered. Again with hindsight, it might have been better to select locations nearer base.

Whilst examining mainly psychiatric care contexts, the study did examine one unit (R1 ward) which was a ward for women with severe learning disabilities requiring the secure care of Rampton Hospital. Whilst showing some interestingly similar characteristics to other care locations, this ward was somewhat untypical; and it is questionable whether the study would not have benefited more by omitting R1 ward, and instead augmenting the internal contexts of acute psychiatric care observed by adding a further mental illness ward.

Finally, few, if any, empirically-based studies in forensic psychiatric nursing care relate to patient outcomes (Hayward, 1986). Whilst such studies are beyond the scope of this study, positive indicators have emerged within it that could well facilitate future outcome research. Nevertheless, the fact that the present study does not address patient outcomes may be regarded as a weakness; though there are equally weighty arguments for considering that attempting such work as part of the present study would have been over-ambitious and rather premature.

Implications for further work

Clinical implications

The growth of individualised nursing care within the study locations is clearly progressing; although much requires to be done before significant increases in resultant quality of nursing care can be achieved. Deficits in care delivery naturally lead to a reduction in quality of care and in quality of life for involved patients. The attendant decrease in task-allocated care behaviours has yet to achieve "critical" frequencies before it differs convincingly from that previously observed in traditional institutional regimes. In some cases, nurses still require persuading that change is a never-ending cycle; and that care patterns must remain dynamic if patients are continually to receive the "best possible" nursing care which the social context can offer.

The relationships that individualised care programmes have helped foster through patient participation in care planning are evident; although much has to be done in connection with staff acquisition of interactional skills. The role of the key nurse, whilst in theory it assists in developing these relationships, gives some cause for concern. Socially compatible "partnerships" and contracting techniques need to be at the forefront when "allocating" patients to nurses; and the effects carefully monitored.

Monitoring of nursing care processes is crucial for care to remain dynamic.

This is not to say that hierarchal checking should be carried out: but rather that there is a distinct need to involve both nursing staff and patients in evaluating what they do. The contemporary, and relatively recent, expectation that nurses should develop a poised, sceptical, questioning and evaluative approach to clinical practice may be especially helpful here.

Although they are on the increase, consumer studies within Rampton Hospital have yet to examine those relationship issues which are vital to the growth of care partnerships. The restriction of patients' freedom of choice is, at the least, an invasion to some degree of their rights to self-determination in terms of everyday nursing care.

Monitoring of clinical practice is crucial to its dynamic growth. Regular reviews involving patients and nursing staff should ideally form a key feature of ward evaluation. Such evaluation would facilitate gradual change in clinical practice, promoting quality of health care; therapeutic nurse-patient relationships; and innovative care practice.

Current low frequencies of individualised and direct patient care are swamped by time devoted to traditional ward routines. Contemporary uncertainties in the nurse's role vis-a-vis therapeutic involvement, and attendant role-abridgement within well-understood "supervisory" modes, need to be overcome if effective therapeutic interventions are to increase. Nursing skills in relation to perception of, and ability to accommodate, patient needs require urgent review to ensure consistent and appropriate care programmes. Similarly, current high frequencies of administrative behaviours on the part of more qualified and experienced nurses indicate the need for effective resource management to enable redirection of such scarce nursing resources.

The balance between theory and security within the Rampton Hospital contexts is of special importance. At the present time, gearing of supervisory care towards "worst-care" scenarios often overrides important therapeutic inputs. Care needs to be more proactive than reactive in nature. Similarly, improvement in nurse-patient communications and relationships would materially serve to improve the calibre of clinical nursing care.

Management implications

Among the study's considerable implications for managers, perhaps most important are the ways in which its findings have been, and can be, used. Managers, and especially ward managers, are in a unique position to implement research findings and influence clinical practice. As well as indicating general quantitative trends, the related methods allow the fine details of contemporary empirical care processes to be evaluated.

Such "fine-grained" details are an extremely valuable resource for managers.

In the climate of quality and cost-effectiveness in relation to health care, knowledge of such details can help facilitate optimal allocation of scarce nursing resources. Thus managers can be materially helped in their central task of ensuring that appropriate nursing skills are made available to meet the needs of individual patients. Such techniques offer a unique opportunity for managers to be central in influencing patient care delivery. They can, as a result, explore various ways in which nurses' time can be freed-up from task-orientated approaches, thus preparing the way for more direct care through approaches such as the nursing process.

The observed "overburden" of nurses with administrative duties, and especially paperwork, needs careful reappraisal by clinical managers to examine to what extent this is taking nurses away from direct patient care. Similarly, they need to examine research findings, including those of the present study, to gain systematic insights into the nature and processes involved in patient care. Such evidence would assist in changing traditional perspectives and allowing innovative thinking in the organisation concerning staffing and the processes of care delivery.

Workforce planning is an essential part of a managers' everyday work routine. Whilst not technically a manpower system, the observational method used in this study has close affinities with nursing activity instruments. The special descriptive features of the ward observation schedule allow more detailed and precise accounts of observed care than is usually the case with such instruments. These should be the first step in workforce planning, which regrettably is often missing in current systems. That is, by assessing the meaning of these descriptive details it is possible to use them to gain the best from current nursing resources.

Educational implications

It is unsure from this study to what extent managers are prepared in terms of understanding the nature and concept of the nursing process model of care delivery. However, indications are that, as with lack of effective training for other nurses, there is still not a full managerial understanding of the potential power of the concept. Clinical managers, being those best placed to influence practice, thus need to be provided with appropriate developmental programmes (Robinson, 1994). Managers will not be in a position to initiate scientific clinical change unless they fully understand the meaning and nature of the concept.

Since all nurses have not yet received formal education in individual care programmes, and considerable resultant deficits were observed in low-scoring care planning documentation, there are clear indications for increasing educational opportunities for all nurses in connection with the nursing process. The data indicated considerable variance in care planning knowledge and skills between the five locations studied. These need systematic review in order to provide appropriate new opportunities in professional development for the nurses concerned.

Whilst the work of Carton (1990) is already contributing to the continuing education of nursing staff in this respect, his customised programme is as yet only available to the limited number of nurses working in units which are voluntary participants in care planning audit and subsequent intervention. Considerable effort is now required in care planning audit on a wider scale; identification of related skills; and, where there are shortfalls, introduction of appropriate strategies to sustain and improve related knowledge and skills. Similarly, such interventions should not be regarded as isolated, one-off experiences. Regular updates and continual monitoring need to take place if the work is to be sustained and impact meaningfully on clinical care.

The nursing process has now been operating to some degree at Rampton Hospital for more than two decades; and the problems noted today are depressingly similar to those encountered shortly after its inception. Earlier formal education was not succeeded by periodic review; or by attempts systematically to involve all nursing staff in its principles; or by attempts to develop or deepen its rather cursory introductory treatment. If contemporary education is to succeed, it must be based on the identified needs of the nursing workforce, rather than simply assuming that provision of various formal courses will cater automatically for their needs. Additionally, systematic and rigorous patient needs assessment, and resultant updating in relation to staff and patient needs, should be carried out.

The present fluctuating occupational climate, with attendant changes in the nursing workforce, do little to develop care practice positively at clinical level. Indeed, the opposite sometimes appears to be the case; and change overburdens nurses with ever more policies and procedures. Such organisational shifts need to be more effectively geared to patient and staff needs; possibly through the commissioning of a systematic review of the effects, both potential and actual, of such changes on patient care.

The increasing paperwork, whilst important, needs continual monitoring to scrutinise its relevance to clinical care. The nursing process has frequently been characterised by practitioners as a paper exercise; and where such attitudes prevail this may indeed become the case. The present study has shown examples of the generalised and often meaningless entries on care plans which this attitude encourages. Nurses need to be convinced of the importance of complete and concise documentation, vital to the assessment and evaluation of care practice.

Extended observational studies Follow-up of clinical observations on other wards would provide each ward with baseline data on patient care. This work is vital if such care is to be improved and a consistent quality of service for patients developed.

Extension of study to women's wards Whilst already yielding some interesting data, R1 ward clearly requires further study; as do other units accommodating women. There are currently approximately 120 female patients within Rampton Hospital. Although some preliminary studies have been carried out in relation to self-harming behaviours on female wards, and R4 ward is the subject of considerable study, women's wards in general have necessarily received scant attention within the contexts of the present study.
There is a pressing need for similar studies to be undertaken within environments caring for women at Rampton Hospital.

Development of outcome measures The study has identified some promising indicators for potential use in the development of patient outcome measures. There is now a need to re-examine the data carefully with a view to developing indices for patient outcome measurement scales. Such outcome measures would significantly support and complement qualitative observational studies, since the latter give precise details regarding the processes of care. Some form of qualitative ordinal evaluation would contribute towards the understanding, description and explanation of a context and a population both of which have been considerably under-studied.

Developing observational studies Whilst confined in the present study to descriptions of nurses' behaviour, the ward observation schedule may also be used for recording behavioural characteristics of patients. This schedule is extremely adaptable due to its descriptive format; and development in this area could be moved forward considerably. Rigorous research using this method could contribute substantially to descriptions of health status and behavioural characteristics of patients being treated within the forensic psychiatric care setting. Such data would provide first-hand knowledge and insights into a considerably under-researched area.

Focused outcome studies The study has already to some extent influenced development of indicators for patient consumerism. Such indicators, whilst giving insights into the quality of life for patients, do little to describe or measure how patients actually get better as a result of therapeutic interventions.

Therefore studies are required to examine patient outcomes; especially in relation to issues surrounding the direct reason for admission to a Special Hospital.

Analogous studies in learning disability One of the limitations of this study was identified as a lack of locations and informants relating to patients with learning disabilities. Whilst showing that there are some similarities within care delivery constructs, much more data are required concerning this important patient group. This is especially so within the female population of Rampton Hospital; and research into these areas is urgently needed.

Interdisciplinary nursing studies This study has briefly indicated some interesting relationships between behavioural patterns of nurses working within forensic, mainstream psychiatric, and general nursing contexts. Though these data are fascinating and possibly indicative, further research is required to establish to what extent similarities hold good; and where the critical differentiae occur.

Nurse-patient relationships Patients pointed out the restrictions in relationships possibly resulting from some interpretation of the role of the key nurse. Given the lack of nurse-initiated interactions, and the general lack of genuinely therapeutic relationships between patients and nurses, systematic review of current interpretations of the role is required. Mention was made earlier of patterns of "overcaring". The assignment of key nurses to patients, with little regard to patients' needs or appropriate nursing skills, could result in such "overcaring", which is a poor preparation for return to the external world. Therefore the process of assigning key nurses; its impacts on patient care; and its therapeutic value, all require systematic review.

Impact of paperwork Paperwork takes up considerable nursing time and reduces time available for potential therapeutic inputs. Paperwork and its related tasks need further research to determine its quality and appropriateness; and to explore how nursing time may best be freed-up for involvement in more direct nursing care.

Educational intervention studies Educational requirements have been frequently cited within this report. In order to improve nurses' knowledge and skills in relation to individual care planning and delivery, a substantial audit of care planning practices, including related documentation and resultant action, needs to be a main feature of the hospital's programme of educational research. Such an audit would be the logical precursor of individual, ward-based programmes of action research, directed towards design and delivery of "customised" teaching and learning packages for the nursing staff concerned.

Impact of changing care ideologies   Organisational change has been considerable within the last decade. Nurses have been faced with profound modifications in ideologies of health care: for example, the advent of nursing process and quality care issues. It is largely unknown what impact, if any, these have had in terms of patient health status. In particular it is not known how, or to what extent, the nursing process model of care delivery actually impacts on the improved health status of patients. This area demands creative and forward-looking outcome research as a matter of urgent priority.

WARD OBSERVATION SCHEDULE

WARD: .... DATE: .... SHEET NO: ....

SHEET STARTED: .... SHEETFINISHED:.....................

1 NS/PT	2 DESCRIPTION OF BEHAVIOUR	3 CODE	4 LOC	5 NO S	6 NO P
	0 1 2 → P N R T A L				
	0 1 2 → P N R T A L				
	0 1 2 → P N R T A L				
	0 1 2 → P N R T A L				

KEY: 0 = indirect care; 1 = group care; 2 = individual care; P=patient-initiated interaction; N=nurse-initiated interaction; R=nurse rejects patients; T=nurse tolerates patient; A=nurse accepts patient. L= language use. Where language is used, one of the following codes should be entered: 1=audible talk; 2=angry talk; 3=negative control; 4=positive control; 5=programmatic talk; 6=explanatory talk; 7=expressions of affection or regard.

Key to observation codes

AS (administrative-supervisory) = non-patient-related discussion or behaviour of an administrative or supervisory nature. Examples include paperwork; answering the telephone; checking stocks or giving instructions.

SP (supervisory-patient) = patient-related discussion or interaction of a supervisory nature. Examples include supervising toileting or bathing; counselling or giving instructions to patients; advising or discussing care.

PS (patient-social) = task-oriented social care of patients unrelated to individual care plans. Examples include saying good morning/goodbye to patients; playing games with, or watching television with, patients.

PF (patient-functional) = general task-oriented physical care of patients, unrelated to individual care plans. Examples include helping patients to get up or to walk; wiping bottoms or noses; washing or drying of patients.

NP (nursing process) = verbal or non-verbal interactions to do with any of the stages of care planning: that is, assessment; care planning; implementation and evaluation. Examples include filling in assessment forms; giving care to patients as prescribed in individual care plans; and evaluating care.

DM (domestic) = non-patient-related discussion or behaviour to do with domestic issues in ward management. Examples include cleaning or polishing floors; washing objects; or clearing away after play sessions.

MS (miscellaneous) = examples of staff discussion or behaviour which do not fit under any of the other descriptive codes; and in which no recognisable nursing element can be found. Examples include chit-chat between staff; eating or drinking; staff in toilet or talking to researcher.

CE (clinical education) = This code refers to all aspects of nurse education to all members of the clinical team. Examples include discussions of ward procedures, updating, carrying out procedures as part of nurse training, lectures or seminars by the ward team or tutors.

AE (assessment explicit), that is, verbal behaviour to do with assessment of an individual patient.

AI (assessment implicit), that is, other behaviour by which assessment of an individual patient is IMPLIED, although not specifically mentioned;

PE (planning explicit), that is, verbal behaviour to do with care planning for an individual patient;

PI (planning implicit), that is, other behaviour by which care planning for an individual patient is IMPLIED, although not specifically mentioned;

IE (implementation explicit), that is, verbal behaviour to do with implementation of nursing care for an individual patient;

II (implementation implicit), that is, other behaviour by which implementation of nursing care for an individual patient is IMPLIED, although not specifically mentioned.

EE (evaluation explicit), that is, verbal behaviour to do with evaluation of nursing care for an individual patient;

EI (evaluation implicit), that is other behaviour by which evaluation of nursing care for an individual patient is IMPLIED, although not specifically mentioned.

Revised behavioural codes

CWP (communication with patient) Any one-to-one communication with a patient, by word or sign, about any topic, other than care plan activity. Examples include, casual conversation, talking a patient through an activity, giving directions to a patient and collecting information from the patient.

CPA (care plan activity) Any verbal or non-verbal behaviour relating to the individual care plan. Examples include, assisting the patient actually carry out an assessment or making an assessment, planning care, implementing the plan, evaluation and completing progress notes.

PTF (patient-functional) Any general, task-orientated, physical care of patients, unrelated to an individual care plan (actually doing things for or assisting patients).

PTS (patient-social) Behaviours relating to task-orientated social care of patients, unrelated to task-orientated social care of patients, unrelated to an individual care plan. Examples include, playing games, watching TV or general chit-chat with patients.

GPT (group therapy) Taking part in, running or acting as co-worker, in a therapy group. These are groups with a direct therapeutic purpose, rather than simply general social groups. Examples include, counselling or anger management groups.

MED (medication) Administering medication, either as part of a medicine round, depot injection or on a PRN basis. Other examples include, reading medicine cards or filling them in.

PSI (patient supervision on the ward) Staff supervision of patients within the ward, but not participating in care plan activity: eg, sitting in the dayroom with patients, moving patients from room to room within the ward, or unlocking a door, seeing a patient through it and locking it again.

CAP (communication with patient): Any verbal behaviour relating to a patient but not actually involving the patient or concerning his/her care plan. Examples include, staff discussions about patient in general terms, or related to his/her health status, with any member of the clinical team.

IWA (in the ward administration): Any discussion, paperwork or other behaviour that contributes to the running of the ward, but not to any individual care plan: eg, filling out menus, meeting visitors, answering general telephone calls, filling in documents or filing them, giving instructions to staff.

DOM (domestic): Behaviours and discussions related to ward domestic arrangements rather than to patients. These may be related to, or involve carrying out ward cleaning or storage of items such as laundry and serving food.

PER (personal): Any verbal or non-verbal behaviours of a personal nature: eg, eating, drinking, going to the toilet, reading the newspaper or general chit-chat unrelated to the ward.

CLE (clinical education): Any discussions or behaviour relating to any aspect of nurse education, involving any member(s) of the nursing team, including students). Examples may include, participating in seminars, ward discussions, nurse- or tutor-led sessions, undertaking tests or other learning experiences.

OWD (off-ward duties): Any behaviour relating to ward management taking place outside the ward. Examples include, collecting drugs from pharmacy, collection of files, taking patients to X-ray or other services.

LOB (level of observation): Any verbal or non-verbal behaviour that relates to the observation, documentation and communication of patients who require close observation. These should include observations that are care-plan related. Examples include level 2 and 3 observations; seclusion; completing related documents; and discussion of such a patient's health status.

NURSING PROCESS RECORDS - DOCUMENTARY ANALYSIS

(SAMPLE CRITERIA)

WARD/DEPARTMENT ....

PATIENT'S NAME ....

DATE OF ANALYSIS ....

INSTRUCTIONS:

Carefully examine ALL nursing records in relation to each patient, with special reference to his care plan(s) and treatment record(s). Then ring the appropriate digit in relation to each item in the following checklist. SCORE ONLY ON INFORMATION ACTUALLY PRESENT IN NURSING RECORDS, UNLESS OTHERWISE INDICATED. Finally, add up and record the total score for each section and the grand total score, and record these at the end of the checklist in the spaces provided. Should any item not be considered relevant, exclude it and subtract its maximum score (3) from the total possible score for that section.

KEY TO CHECKLIST:

NO RECORD (NR): indicates that the item cannot be found in any of the documents examined. (ie, NO ATTEMPT MADE - SCORE 0)

PARTIAL RECORD (PR): indicates that a relatively brief and uninformative mention of the item can be found. (ie, SLIGHT ATTEMPT MADE - SCORE 1)

INCOMPLETE RECORD (IR): indicates that, although an appreciable attempt has been made, the item is recorded in an unclear or ambiguous manner. (ie, FAIR ATTEMPT MADE - SCORE 2)

COMPLETE RECORD (CR): indicates that a clear, detailed and informative mention of the item can be found. (ie, GOOD ATTEMPT MADE - SCORE 3).

NO	ITEM:	NR	PR	IR	CR
	A. ASSESSMENT PHASE				
1	An assessment was made on admission, prior to implementing the NP.	0	1	2	3
2	There is a record of discussion(s) involving patient, family and nursing staff all meeting together.	0	1	2	3
3	The patient's previous history (ie, relevant details prior to admission is recorded.	0	1	2	3
4	Attempt(s) to foster trust and a positive atmosphere for the patient are clear from the notes.	0	1	2	3

NO	ITEM:	NR	PR	IR	CR
	B. PLANNING PHASE				
1	The patient's needs or problems (and, when appropriate, his strengths) are clearly indicated in the written care plan.	0	1	2	3
2	The nursing objective(s) are clearly stated in the written care plan.	0	1	2	3
3	A clear and precise plan of action is given in the written care plan.	0	1	2	3
4	Each need and expected outcome in achieving the therapeutic goal(s) is clearly specified step-by-step in the written care plan.	0	1	2	3

NO	ITEM:	NR	PR	IR	CR
	C. IMPLEMENTATION PHASE				
1	A nurse is allocated to care for this individual patient.	0	1	2	3
2	This nurse-patient contact is maintained each day as far as is possible.	0	1	2	3
3	There is evidence of face-to-face inter-shift communication with regard to this care plan.	0	1	2	3
4	Written progress reports appear relevant to this care plan.	0	1	2	3

NO	ITEM:	NR	PR	IR	CR
	D. EVALUATION PHASE				
1	A definite date for evaluation is entered into the care plan.	0	1	2	3
2	Evaluations of the patient's progress have been recorded.	0	1	2	3
3	Effects of nursing intervention have been recorded.	0	1	2	3
4	Nursing actions have clearly been modified when appropriate.	0	1	2	3

ANNEXE C

PATIENT GUIDED INTERVIEW SCHEDULE

WARD/DEPARTMENT ....

PATIENT CODE ....

DATE .... TIME STARTED................. TIME FINISHED.............

SECTION A: EMPLOYMENT AND RECREATIONAL INTERESTS

A1   PREVIOUS EMPLOYMENT

Q: Could we start by you telling me what sorts of jobs you had before come here?

PROBES: Did you work anywhere? (IF YES) What type of job did you do? Who did you work for? Did you enjoy the work? (IF NO) Haven't you had any jobs at all? What type of work would you like to do?

A2   PRESENT EMPLOYMENT

Q: Do you work in any of the shops or departments here?

PROBES: Which shops do you work in? What do you do in the shops? Do you enjoy working there? (IF YES) Why do you like working there? (IF NO) Why do you say that you don't like working there? Is there anywhere where you feel you would like to work? (IF YES) Why do you think you would like working there?

A3   RECREATIONAL INTERESTS

Q: How do you like to spend your spare time?

PROBES: Do you have any hobbies or something that you like to do? What are those? When do you do that? Do you do it on the ward? Is there anything that you would like to do in your spare time? (IF YES) What is that? Why would you like to do that?

A4   RECREATION INTERACTION

Q: Do you ever play any of the ward games, such as table tennis?

PROBES: (IF YES) What games do you play? Who plays with you? Who joins in? Do you win? Are there competitions or is it just for fun? (IF NO) Why don't you play any ward games? Are there any that you would like to play? What are those? Why do you think you would like to play that game/those games?

SECTION B: PATIENT PERCEPTIONS OF CARE

B1   NURSE/PATIENT RELATIONSHIP

Q: I notice today that there are quite a few nurses on duty. Is there always a staff available if you need to talk to him/her?

PROBES: (IF YES) Do you go to the same nurse all the time? Is there a nurse who seems to help you more than the others? (IF NO) When is there no one around to talk to you? Do you ever have problems in contacting staff? (IF S0) When? What are they?

B2   NURSE/PATIENT COMMUNICATION

Q: Do you find that the nurses have time to talk to you?

PROBES: Do they sit down with you and chat? (IF YES) What do you talk about? Do you talk about your future? (IF NO) Surely they must talk to you sometimes? Can you remember what you talk about? Who else talks to you? Do nurses come to chat to you or do you have to go to the nurses?

B3   PATIENT INVOLVEMENT IN CARE

Q: Does anybody ever ask you to talk about your care on this ward?

PROBES: Do the nurses tell you about your care? (IF YES) Can you remember what they told you? Did they ask what you felt about it? Have you ever filled in forms or papers? Can you remember what they were about? (IF NO) Has anybody said anything to you about what is happening? Who was that? Are you invited to ward meetings? Who is there? What do you talk about?

B4   CARE NEEDS

Q: Do you think you should help decide your own care whilst on this ward?

PROBES: (IF YES) What care do you think you should receive? How would you like to be involved? How would you like to be helped? Who would you like to help you? (IF NO) What do you feel about that? I mean, do you feel you should have some say in your own care?

B5   DIRECT CARE

Q: Are there any areas that the nurses are helping you with?

PROBES: Are the nurses on here helping you learn anything? Is there anything with which you would like a little help from the nurses? (IF YES) What are they helping you with? How are they helping you? Does anyone else help you? (IF NO) Are you sure that NOBODY ever helps you at all?

B6   PERCEPTIONS OF HOSPITAL/WARD

Q: Do you have any feelings about this ward?

PROBES: I mean what do you think about this ward? What are the things you like about it? Why is that? Is there anything not so good about this ward? Could anything be improved? Why is that? How could it be improved? Does it affect you? In what way?

SECTION C: FAMILY AND OTHER OUTSIDE CONTACT

C1   SOCIAL CONTACT

Q: Does anyone come to visit you?

PROBES: Do your family or friends come to visit you? Who comes to visit you? Do they come very often? (IF THEY DO VISIT) do they ever speak to the ward nurses? Would you like them to? Is there any way that you think your visitors could help? (IF NO VISITORS) Would you like someone to visit you? Who would you like to visit you? How do you think it would help you?

ANNEXE D

NURSING STAFF GUIDED INTERVIEW SCHEDULE

WARD/DEPARTMENT: .... STAFF CODE: ....

STAFF GRADE: .... DATE: ....

TIME STARTED: .... TIME FINISHED: ....

SECTION A: BACKGROUND INFORMATION
A1   AGE GROUP

     18-30   31-40   41-50   51-60
     (please circle as appropriate)

A2   EDUCATIONAL BACKGROUND

     Type of school attended:
     Grammar   Secondary Modern   Comprehensive

     Other ....

A3   GENERAL EDUCATIONAL QUALIFICATIONS
     (please specify below, with date(s) obtained)

A4   EMPLOYMENT PRIOR TO NURSING
     (please specify below, with dates)

     OCCUPATION   FROM   TO

SECTION B: PROFESSIONAL BACKGROUND AND PERCEIVED ROLE
B1   NURSE TRAINING

     SCHOOL OF NURSING   DATES

B2   NURSING QUALIFICATIONS

     QUALIFICATION   DATE

B3   PREVIOUS NURSE EXPERIENCE
Q: Could we start with a few questions about your own nursing experience: What had you done in nursing so far, before working on this ward?

B4   EXPERIENCE ON PRESENT WARD
Q: How long have you worked on this ward?

B5   WORK PREFERENCES
Q: Is there any type of ward or area where you specially like to work?

B6   NON-PREFERRED AREAS
Q: Is there any type of ward/area where you don't particularly like to work?

B7   PERCEIVED CAREER DEVELOPMENT
Q: How do you see your future career developing in nursing?

B8   TRAINING/EDUCATIONAL NEEDS
Q: Do you feel you would benefit from any kind of in-service education or training courses?

B9   PERSONAL SKILLS
Q: What would you say are your main strengths as a nurse?

B10   INVOLVEMENT WITH PATIENTS
Q: Do you think that, nowadays, nurses are becoming MORE involved or LESS involved with patients?

SECTION C: WARD/UNIT CARE PLANNING AND COMMUNICATION
C1   TYPE(S) OF PATIENTS
Q: Perhaps we would now move on to talk a bit about the ward/unit and patients.... Can you tell me a bit about the (various) type(s) of patient you nurse on this ward?

C2   PATIENT NEEDS
Q: What do you feel are their main nursing needs?

C3   WARD/UNIT AIMS
Q: Do you have any general aims for this ward/unit?

C4   PERCEIVED REALISM OF AIMS
Q: (IF YES TO C3) How close would you say you come to achieving those general aims?

C5   RELEVANCE OF INDIVIDUAL CARE PLANS
Q: Speaking generally, how relevant would you say the individual care plans are to helping the patients solve their problems?

C6   PATIENT AWARENESS OF CARE PLAN
Q: Do you patients know that they are on some kind of nursing care plan?

C7   PATIENT INVOLVEMENT IN CARE PLANNING
Q: Are you patients ever involved in deciding on goals for their own care plans?

C8   DISCIPLINARY INVOLVEMENT IN CARE PLANNING
Q: Who actually gets involved when you are deciding on the content of patient care plans?

C9   INVOLVEMENT OF OTHER AREAS/DEPARTMENTS
Q: Are you care plans confined to periods when the patient is actually in the ward/unit?

C10   COMMUNICATING THE CARE PLAN
Q: When starting or running a care plan, how do you make sure that all the other staff who will need to be involved know about it?

C11   COMMUNICATIVE VALUE OF CARE PLANS
Q: Do you think that care plans THEMSELVES can influence communication in any way?

C12   PRACTICAL OUTCOMES
Q: Do you feel that care planning affects individual care on this ward/unit?

C13   STANDARDS OF CARE
Q: How do you ensure that patients on this ward receive effective nursing care?

SECTION D: GENERAL PERCEPTIONS OF THE NURSING PROCESS
D1   DEFINING THE NURSING PROCESS
Q: Perhaps we could move on to think about the Nursing Process a little more generally now .... What do the words "Nursing Process" mean to you?

D2 PERSONAL REACTIONS TO THE NURSING PROCESS
Q: What do you, personally, feel about the Nursing Process?

D3 POTENTIAL ADVANTAGES
Q: What do you think its main advantages could be?

D4 POTENTIAL DISADVANTAGES
Q: What do you think its main disadvantages could be?

D5 INTRODUCING THE NURSING PROCESS
Q: Can you remember how the Nursing Process was first introduced to your ward?

D6 INITIAL PERCEPTIONS
Q: Can you remember your feelings and impressions at the time when the Nursing Process was first introduced?

D7 COLLEAGUES' PERCEPTIONS
Q: How do you think other nurses felt about it at that time?

D8 PREPARATION FOR THE NURSING PROCESS
Q: Was any preparation for use of the Nursing Process provided for ward/unit staff?

D9 UNDERLYING PRINCIPLES
Q: Was any training provided in knowledge and skills necessary to carry out Nursing Process - such as communication skills, or theory of Nursing Process, for example?

D10 CURRENT OPERATIONAL STATUS
Q: How do you feel the Nursing Process is operating now?

D11 COLLEAGUES' OPINIONS OF CURRENT OPERATIONAL STATUS
Q: I know it is difficult to speak for others, but what do you feel is the general attitude of Rampton nurses towards the Nursing Process, now that it is established and running?

D12 PLANNING THE CHANGE
Q: With hindsight, do you think that enough care and thought went into introducing the Nursing Process when it first appeared?

D13   MULTIDISCIPLINARY INVOLVEMENT
Q: How involved do you think members of other disciplines (such as medicine and psychology, for example) should be in care planning for your patients?

D14   STRUCTURE OF NURSING CARE PLAN
Q: There are a number of different models of a care plan in use right now. Could you describe the stages of the type of care plan you are familiar with?

D15   PAPERWORK
Q: What do you think are the advantages and disadvantages of the paperwork involved in Nursing Process?

D16   COURSES ON NURSING PROCESS
Q: Apart from the sort of preparation we've been talking about, have you ever attended any courses on the Nursing Process?

SECTION E: MONITORING CARE

E1   MONITORING THE NURSING PROCESS
Q: Now that the Nursing Process has been implemented here for quite some time, do you feel there is still a need for somebody to monitor it?

E2   QUALITY CARE
Q: Do you think nurses can help improve care services to patients?

E3   MISCELLANEOUS ISSUES
Q: Finally, is there anything else - any other issue which you'd like to raise just before we finish?

FOR NIGHT STAFF ONLY:
E4   INVOLVEMENT OF NIGHT STAFF
Q: What do you feel about the use of the Nursing Process on night duty?

ANNEXE E

SELECTED READING LIST

Argyle, M (1973): Social Encounters: Readings into Social Interaction. Middlesex: Penguin Books.

Berger, P L and Luckman, T (1967): The Social Construction of Reality: A Treatise in the Sociology of Knowledge. Norwich: Penguin.

Chalmers, A F (1976): What is this thing called Science? An assessment of the Nature and Status of Science. Milton Keynes: The Open University Press.

Douglas, M (1980): Evans-Pritchard. Glasgow: William Collins Sons and Co Ltd.

English National Board (1988): Managing Change in Education: An ENB Work Package London: English National Board.

Fawcett, J and Downs, F S (1986): The Relationships of Theory and Research. Norwalk, Connecticut: Appleton-Century-Crofts.

Goffman, E (1971): Relations in Public: Microstudies of the Public Order. Middlesex: Penguin Books.

Guiraud, P (1975): Semiology. London: Routledge and Kegan Paul.

Harre, R and Secord, P F (1972): The Explanation of Social Behaviour. Oxford: Basil Blackwell.

Hinder, R A (1982): Ethology. Glasgow: William Collins Sons & Co Ltd.

Kelly, A V (1986): Knowledge of Curricular Planning. London: Harper and Row.

Leach, E (1970): Levi-Strauss. London: Wm Collins and Co Ltd.

Leach, E (1982): Social Anthropology. Glasgow: William Collins Sons and Co Ltd.

Luckman, T (1978): Phenomenology and Sociology. Middlesex: Penguin Books.

Munhall, P L and Oiler, C J (1986): Nursing Research: A Qualitative Perspective. Norwalk, Connecticut, Appleton-Century-Crofts.

O'Brient, D, Clinton, M and Cruddace, H (1985): Managing and Mismanaging Change: The Case of the Nursing Process. Paper presented at Annual Conference at the RCN Research Society, University of Nottingham, March 1985.

O'Conner, D J (1957): An Introduction to the Philosophy of Education. London: Routledge and Kegan Paul.

Peters, R S ed (1967): The Concept of Education. London: Routledge and Kegan Paul.

Torres, G (1986): Theoretical Foundations of Nursing. Norwalk, Connecticut: Appleton-Century-Crofts.

RESEARCH, PUBLICATIONS AND CONFERENCE PAPERS

Completed Research:

A Pilot Study of the Ward Interaction Observation Schedule. Wakefield Health Authority (1987).

Staff Preferences in Continuing Education. Rampton Hospital (1987).

Variables Influencing Response Rates in Questionnaires. Rampton Hospital (1988).

Measuring Quality Care in a Special Hospital: An Approach through the Nursing Process. Diploma in Research (with special commendation) Bournemouth Polytechnic/Rampton Hospital (1988).

An Evaluation of Patient Assessment Models and their Research Projects. Rampton Hospital (1991).

What Happens to Research Reports? An Evaluation of ENB 870 Research Projects. Rampton Hospital (1991).

Patient Visiting: The Consumer View. Rampton Hospital, (1992). Achievements and Opportunities: A Review of Rampton Hospital Community Liaison Service: Rampton Hospital (1992).

Patient Choice and Privacy. Rampton Hospital (1993).

Current PhD study, Developing Clinical Quality Indicators in Psychiatric Nursing. Rampton Hospital/Anglia College (1994).

Developing the Contribution of Research in Nursing: An Evaluation towards a Strategy for Research and Development. SHSA (1994).

Ongoing Research:

A Survey of Research Priorities within the Special Hospitals Service Authority. SHSA (1994).

Research in Nursing: Where are We? Rampton Hospital (1994).

Publications: As well as the publications listed below a number of articles have been written for hospital research journals and bulletins.

Response Rates in Questionnaires. Senior Nurse, November/December 1989, Vol 9, No 10, pp 25-26.

Two Decades of "The Process". Senior Nurse, February, 1990, Vol 10, No 2, pp 4-6.

Qualitative Analysis of Quality Care. Senior Nurse, July 1990, Vol 10, No 7, pp 21-25.

An Innovative Approach to Teaching the Nursing Process. Nursing Standard. November 1990, Vol 5, No 22, pp 30-32.

Nursing Research at Rampton Hospital: An Overview 1991-92. Research News, Rampton Hospital, 1992, Issue 4, pp 5-6.

Hand-held Computers in Audit Data Collection and Analysis. News in brief, in Journal of Nursing Management (1992).

Use of Hand-held Terminals for Data Capture within Health Care Systems. Journal of Nursing Management, Feb 1993, 1, pp 47-49.

Hand-held Computers in Clinical Audit. Senior Nurse, May/June 1993, Vol 13, No 3, pp 14-17.

Direct Downloading: A Route to Rapid Feedback. Quality Connection, July/August 1993, Vol 2, Issue 1, pp 1-2.

Computer Based Research: Hand-held Computers in Data Collection. Special Hospitals Service Authority Journal, Special Edition. Summer 1993, issue 2, pp 3 and 8.

Forensic Psychiatric Nursing: An Evolving Community Role. First International Conference on Community Health Nursing Research. September, 1993, p 121. Health Promotion, Illness and Injury Prevention. Edmonton, Canada, Edmonton Board of Health.

Computerised Observational Audit. In Managing Information for the Benefit of Patients (1993). Weybridge: BJHC Books.

Computerised Observational Care Audit, article accepted for Journal of Quality Assurance.

Developing the Contribution of Research in Nursing: An Evaluation Towards a Strategy for Research and Development. Ashworth Hospital reprographics department (1994). London, SHSA.

The Use of Hand-held Computers in Clinical Audit Data Capture. Article accepted for the DOH Quality Initiatives book due to be published in Spring 1994.

Qualitative Design and Analysis of Care. Article under review by Journal of Nursing Management.

What happens to Research Reports? Article under review by Journal of Nursing Management.

Conference Papers/Presentations: Most conference presentations have resulted in published abstracts often lodged with Department of Health library.

Development of the Ward Interaction Observation Schedule. Stanley Royd Hospital, October 1987.

Curricular Implications of Individualised Care in Forensic Nursing. 6th Annual Research in Education Conference, San Francisco, USA, January 1988.

Evaluative Study of the Nursing Process in a Special Hospital. "A Process for Care", 1st Annual Research Conference, Nursing Research Interest Group Mersey Region (Invited Speaker), March 1988.

Foundation Studies in Quality Care. Inaugural Research Conference, Rampton Hospital, Retford, Notts, June 1988.

Practitioner Research in Action. 7th Annual Research in Education Conference, San Francisco, USA, January 1989.

Measuring Quality Care in a Special Hospital: An Approach through the Nursing Process. Multidisciplinary Research Interest Group, Rampton Hospital, Retford, Notts. March 1989.

Taking Research into the 21st Century. Research Seminar, Rampton Hospital, Retford, Notts. June 1989.

Developing Quality Assurance Measures: Its Implications for Mental Handicap People. Poster given at Quality through Partnership and Practice conference, Society for Mental Handicap, Nottingham, November 1989.

Measuring Quality Care: A Developing Qualitative Approach. National Association for Quality Assurance. Malvern. November 1989, invited speaker.

A Qualitative Approach to the Measurement of Quality Care. International Quality Assurance Conference, Stockholm, Sweden, June 17-19 1990.

What Happens to Research Reports? An Evaluation of ENB 870 Research Projects. "Research in Nursing Practice" National Research Conference, Rampton Hospital, June 20, 1990.

Measuring Quality Care: An Approach through the Nursing Process. National Care Planning Group Conference, Kingsclere Centre, Basingstoke District Hospital, Berks. August 15, 1990 (invited speaker).

Developing Clinical Quality Indicators. Poster given at Birmingham National Quality Exhibition, 1991.

Research and its Implications for Quality. South Thames School of Nursing. National Research and Quality Conference, Dartford, May 1991.

Observational Measures as Indicators for Quality. Rampton Hospital National Research Conference, June 1991.

Qualitative Measurement of the Process of Care. 1st National QUAN Conference, Oxford University, July 1991.

Developing Clinical Quality Indicators in Psychiatric Nursing. Bournemouth University 1st National Quality Conference. September, 1991.

Developing Hand-held Computers for use in Clinical Audit Data Collection. Department of Health Quality Conference. February, 1992.

The Advantages of Qualitative Approaches to the Measurement of Quality. Psychiatric Nursing Audit Project, Newcastle University, May 1992.

Documentary and Observational Audit Measures. Health Sector of Her Majesties Prison Service, Home Office, London. Invited speaker, September 1992.

The Use of Hand-held Computers for Data Capture in Clinical Audit. National Quality Exhibition, Nottingham General Hospital, February 1993. Invited speaker.

Qualitative Analysis of Patient Care Using Hand-held Computers for Data collection. St James University Hospital, March 1993, invited speaker.

Hand-held Computers in Observational Audit Data collection, 10th International Society for Quality Assurance, Maastricht, Netherlands, June 23, 1993.

Hand-held Computers for Data Capture in Clinical Audit. 3rd National Quality Assurance Conference, Heriot-Watt University, Edinburgh. Edinburgh, July 20, 1993.

Developing Clinical Quality Indicators in Psychiatric Nursing. Institute of Psychiatry, invited speaker, November 1993.

Computerised Observational Care Audit. British Computer Society for Nursing, Annual National Conference. Invited speaker, November 1993.

Research Data Collection and Analysis using Hand-held Computers. Clinical Audit Conference, NEC Birmingham, Department of Health, 1994.

Developing Clinical Quality Indicators in Psychiatric Nursing. RCN Research Society Conference, Hull, April 1994.

INDUCTION COURSE FOR NURSE-OBSERVERS

PRE-COURSE QUESTIONNAIRE

COURSE MEMBER'S NAME ....

The purpose of this questionnaire is to help you and your tutors to identify your individual objectives within the course. Please check each item as follows:

RING LETTER A beside any item which you feel you already know COMPLETELY or have already achieved COMPLETELY before coming on the course.

RING LETTER B beside any item which you feel you know PARTIALLY but not COMPLETELY, or have achieved PARTIALLY but not COMPLETELY, before coming on the course.

RING LETTER C beside any item which you don't already know or haven't yet achieved (or have only partially learned or achieved) prior to coming on the course, but which you would like to know or achieve COMPLETELY by the end of the course.

RING LETTER D beside any item which you don't already know COMPLETELY, or haven't already achieved COMPLETELY before coming on the course, and which you feel it would be difficult to know or achieve COMPLETELY by the end of the course, but which you would like to course to prepare you to achieve AT A LATER DATE.

ITEM	DESCRIPTION	A	B	C	D
A:	INTRODUCTORY				
1	Define "observation"	A	B	C	D
2	Describe types of observation	A	B	C	D
3	Discuss relation between observation and scientific theory(ies)	A	B	C	D

4	Explain logical steps in constructing an observation instrument	A	B	C	D
5	Illustrate these stages by reference to Rampton pilot instruments	A	B	C	D
6	Identify main practical NEEDS in carrying out an observational study	A	B	C	D
7	Identify main practical PROBLEMS in carrying out an observational study	A	B	C	D
8	Explain main factors to consider in organising observations	A	B	C	D
9	Illustrate these organisational factors with reference to the Rampton pilot study	A	B	C	D
10	Identify THREE psychiatric/MH studies in which observational studies were used	A	B	C	D

B   METHODS OF QUALITATIVE ANALYSIS

11	Identify THREE recent qualitative studies in psychiatric/MH care	A	B	C	D
12	Describe the technique(s) used in ONE such study	A	B	C	D
13	Discuss methods and techniques of quantitative analysis	A	B	C	D
14	Discuss methods and techniques of qualitative analysis	A	B	C	D
15	Describe strengths and weaknesses of quantitative/qualitative techniques	A	B	C	D
16	Explain how observation contributes to qualitative studies	A	B	C	D

211

17	Describe ONE method of using the computer in qualitative analysis	A	B	C	D
18	Define "quality assurance"	A	B	C	D
19	Distinguish between QUALITATIVE studies and QUALITY ASSURANCE studies	A	B	C	D
20	Summarise the PURPOSES for which qualitative studies may be carried out	A	B	C	D

C   DESIGNING OBSERVATIONAL INSTRUMENTS

21	Identify THREE essential characteristics of an effective observation instrument	A	B	C	D
22	Tell how to assemble a suitable "item pool"	A	B	C	D
23	Give examples drawn from a suitable "item pool"	A	B	C	D
24	Tell how to develop a schedule (or manual) of observations to be made	A	B	C	D
25	Describe TWO methods of selecting a sample for an observation study	A	B	C	D
26	Define "validity"	A	B	C	D
27	Describe the setting-up of a validity pilot study	A	B	C	D
28	Explain the purpose of "item analysis"	A	B	C	D
29	Define "reliability"	A	B	C	D
30	Describe ONE method of reliability testing	A	B	C	D

D　　USING OBSERVATIONAL INSTRUMENTS

31	Define "observational protocol"	A	B	C	D
32	Describe use of the documentary analytic checklist	A	B	C	D
33	Demonstrate ability to use the documentary analytic checklist	A	B	C	D
34	Demonstrate ability to carry out an observational sequence using the documentary analytic checklist	A	B	C	D
35	Describe use of the ward observation sheet	A	B	C	D
36	Demonstrate ability to use the ward observation sheet	A	B	C	D
37	Demonstrate ability to carry out an observational sequence using the ward observation sheet	A	B	C	D
38	Describe organisation and carrying out of a fieldwork session	A	B	C	D
39	Demonstrate ability to STORE AND RETRIEVE observational data effectively	A	B	C	D
40	Demonstrate ability to ANALYSE observational data effectively	A	B	C	D

INDUCTION COURSE FOR NURSE-OBSERVERS

POST-COURSE QUESTIONNAIRE

COURSE MEMBER'S NAME ....

The purpose of this questionnaire is to help you and your tutors to identify exactly what you have learned or achieved during the course, and what remains to be learned or achieved in the future.

SAME QUESTIONS AS FOR PRE-COURSE QUESTIONNAIRE APPLY TO THIS QUESTIONNAIRE

INDUCTION FOR NURSE OBSERVERS: NOTES ON PRE-COURSE
QUESTIONNAIRE FOR GUIDANCE OF TUTORS

A   INTRODUCTORY:

1. OBSERVATION is the act of obtaining data by direct inspection of the
phenomenon under study.

2. Types of observation described should include PARTICIPANT, SEMI-
PARTICIPANT,   NON-PARTICIPANT,   STRUCTURED   AND
UNSTRUCTURED.

3. The discussion should show how what is observed relates directly to the
theory underlying the observer's approach.   For example, behaviourist
researchers are likely to be interested in FREQUENCIES of specific
behaviours; where phenomenological researchers would be more likely to be
interested in TYPOLOGIES of social response and their qualitative
characteristics, rather that in their frequency of occurrence.   However
rudimentary, the theory always undergirds the type of observation undertaken.

4.   The logical stages involved here include: (1) an INTUITIVE
HYPOTHESIS concerning what is occurring; (2) initial protocol (3)
OPERATIONALISATION of the observations, ie, turning them into
observable units; (4) construction of a viable OBSERVATION SCHEDULE.

6. Main practical needs in observation include: (1) an appropriate observation
venue; (2) relevant field collaboration; (3) a viable observation protocol; (4)
trained observers; (5) access to a suitable sample drawn from the venue; (6)
collaboration of the sample members; (7) ethical analysis and approval of the
enterprise; (8) necessary management approval.

7. The main practical problems encountered in carrying out an observational
study include: (1) ensuring the suitability and availability of an appropriate
venue; (2) effective operationalisation of what is to be observed; (3) ensuring
the validity of the observations in terms of what is to be discovered; (4)
ensuring the inter-rater reliability of the observations; (5) selecting an
appropriate sample; (6) minimising or preferably eliminating observer biases
in the study.

8. The main organisational factors in observation studies include: (1) ensuring an adequate and suitable spread of observations across the working day; (2) ensuring an appropriate variety of situations to be observed; (3) ensuring a rotation of subject types; (4) where appropriate, selecting appropriate observation sequences for detailed examination; (5) guarding against observer vigilance fatigue; (6) arranging for appropriate inter-observer reliability checks.

10. Three psychiatric studies where observational techniques were used include, (eg) (1) ERVING GOFFMAN'S study of asylums; (2) the study by ROSENHAMS called "On being sane in insane places"; (3) observational elements in the two studies by D F S CORMACK called "Psychiatric Nursing Observed" and Psychiatric Nursing Revisited". Three mental handicap studies in which observational techniques were used include, (eg) (1) "Patterns of Residential Care" by KING, RAYNES and TIZARD (1972); (2) The study "Working with Parents - a behavioural approach" by COLIN PRYOR (1973); the study of cue-salience in retardate learning patterns by SINSON and WETHERICK (1972).

B   METHODS OF QUALITATIVE ANALYSIS

11. (Three recent psychiatric and mental handicap studies to be identified from the literature)

12. (one set of methods and techniques from the selected studies to be examined in detail)

13. The main methods and techniques used in quantitative analysis include (1) subscription to the proposition that the phenomena under study may be described numerically in a meaningful way; (2) the use of numerical techniques to illustrate underlying unities or nomothetic characteristics of the phenomena under study; (3) use of statistical concepts and graphic or tabular presentations to describe the phenomena; (4) reliance on probability theory in assessing the likelihood of occurrence of specific phenomena by chance alone. Quantitative analysis thus relies heavily on the graphical presentation of distributions of scores and various associated techniques including (eg) pie/bar charts; measures of central tendency and dispersion; variance within the distribution(s); and various correlation and regression techniques. The classical quantitative method is the laboratory experiment, which relies on control and experimental groups to assess the contribution to the phenomena of one or more independent variables.

14. By contrast, the methods and techniques of qualitative analysis are largely concerned with semantic descriptions of phenomena; and in order to obtain such descriptions a variety of techniques is used, including (eg) (1) various self-report techniques, either unstructured or in the form of questionnaires; (2) so-called "documents of life" (Plummer, K); (3) specially requested journals or event diaries; (4) unstructured or structured interviews. Generally speaking, users of qualitative techniques subscribe to the proposition that, if one wishes to know what an individual thinks about a particular issue, the best to do is ask him or her directly. However, this approach is disputed by nomothetic scientists, who affirm that such techniques can never be wholly unaffected by the distortion of introspection. As C S Lewis puts it, introspection is "... like looking at yourself in a mirror to see what you look like when you're NOT looking at yourself in a mirror!"

15. The strengths of quantitative techniques include: (1) simplicity and brevity of description; (2) lend themselves readily to categorisation and graphic description; (3) are regarded as being capable of producing generalisable findings in the sphere of social science. However, according to some authorities, their disadvantages include: (1) tendency to distortion or deformation of data in order to fit it into predetermined categories; (2) an excessively simplistic approach to the description of social phenomena, which its critics regard as being infinitely more complex than rather simplistic descriptions, offered in terms of one or two independent and/or dependent variables, allow for; (3) its tendency (slightly to misquote WITTGENSTEIN) to "... the bewitchment of the senses by means of numbers", to give a sense of pseudo-respectability to such findings.
Moving on to techniques or qualitative analysis, its strengths include: (1) relative flexibility of method as compared with quantitative experimental techniques; (2) a relatively poised and sceptical attitude towards what may be the rather simplistic findings produced by quantitative analysis; (3) the capacity to switch strategies, either of data collection or analysis, during the progress of the study itself. Conversely, the weaknesses of qualitative analysis include; (1) its relative imprecision; (2) a tendency to lack of generalisability in its findings; (3) the relative "softness" of the measurement involved; (4) an uncomfortable shift of locus of control from the researcher to the research context itself.

16. The contribution of observational techniques to qualitative studies includes: (1) contribution of an additional validational element to supplement verbal accounts; (2) the provision of further cross-validational data by means of which the researcher is enabled to compare his/her own perceptions of the research context and problem with those of the informant(s); (3) the advantage of

looking directly at the research context, rather than seeing it exclusively through the eyes of other observers; (4) the possibility of comparison of structured observations obtained from the research context with those obtained from other similar or analogous contexts.

17. The computer contributes to qualitative analysis in a variety of ways, including (eg): (1) provision of word processing for verbal accounts and report preparation; (2) the production of rapid statistics from frequency counts; (3) the use of graphic facilities in summarising codified behaviour; (4) the use of statistical tests of probability where these are appropriate to the data concerned.

18. In health care contexts, the term QUALITY ASSURANCE refers to various studies monitoring the quality of care to ensure that certain stipulated standards are achieved. Such standards may relate to clinical, management or educational aspects of health care. Characteristically, the process of quality assurance is concerned with the structures, processes and outcomes of health care.

19. Here the essential distinction between qualitative studies and quality assurance studies is that qualitative studies operate in a much wider context; and may be concerned with many factors other than simply quality assurance; though they may contribute significantly to quality assurance studies.

20. Some of the purposes for which qualitative studies may be carried out include (eg) (1) to obtain an account of the perceptions and opinions of the individuals involved in health care, either as professionals or recipients; (2) to describe the structural properties of that care, eg, in terms of facilitative management and/or educational structures; (3) to describe the process of care itself, as delivered to the patient/client by the professional; (4) to describe or discuss outcomes both in clinical/professional terms and in terms of consumer satisfaction; (5) to gain contextual lessons to help in the development of future models of care.

C   DESIGNING OBSERVATIONAL INSTRUMENTS

21. Three essential characteristics of an effective observational instrument include: (1) simplicity of structure; (2) clarify of explanatory language; (3) feasibility of use in the practical research context.

22. In this item reference is made to the "think-tank" approach, in which members of a specially well-informed professional group, or of a patient/client

group with special experience of this area of health care, are requested either to write, or comment upon, items intended to contribute to a valid item pool, to assist in the construction of the research instrument.

23. Here course members are given the option of identifying items from a number of appropriate item pools; including those used (eg) for Psychiatric Audit (Hurst and Howard); Psychiatric Monitor; Julia Brooking's Nursing Process Audit; or the documentary analytic checklist used in the pilot phase of the current Rampton study.

24. Here reference is made to the logic of developing an observational instrument, starting with the intuitive hypothesis; continuing with the carrying-out of unstructured global observations, in order to a "feel" for the research context and problem; then letting the mind play over the pool of unstructured observations, with a view to developing an organising structure under which further, more systematic observations may be carried out. The logic continues with development of this structure (with particular reference to item codes); the selection of specific codes for further study; and the development of a detailed schedule or manual identifying all types of behaviour subsumable under each of the various codes, in order to make subsequent coding as unambiguous as possible.

25. There are numerous methods of selecting a sample for an observational study. Classically, a distinction is drawn between PROBABILITY and NON-PROBABILITY SAMPLING (the latter also sometimes known as "purposive" or "opportunity" sampling). In practical terms, the sample drawn for an observational study is unlikely to be a genuine probability sample; and much more likely to be one of the various non-probability samples, including (eg) a PURPOSIVE sample selected from a specific context with a specific objective in view; an OPPORTUNITY sample drawn from situations which are geographically close to the researcher, or which in other ways present optimal conditions for data collection; a SNOWBALL sample in which small numbers of cases rapidly lead on to others; (add to these definitions of CLUSTER SAMPLE and STRATIFIED sample).

26. The VALIDITY of an instrument is the degree of effectiveness with which it tells us what we want to know, ie, its efficiency in generating valid data for purposes of the study.

27. The classic method of setting up a validity pilot for a specific research instrument is to refer it to a validation sample (or validation panel) of specially

knowledgeable clinicians and/or academics (or, indeed, patients or clients) for purposes of obtaining their opinions regarding the face, content and construct validity of the instrument. Course members should be able to discuss practical methods of setting up such a study.

28. ITEM ANALYSIS may be defined as an attempt to ensure the predictive validity of individual items included in a specific scale or instrument, in relation to the predictive validity of all the other items. An item so analyzed may be considered inappropriate for inclusion if it is a low, or non-predictor, in terms of the general predictive index provided by the instrument as a whole. However, such is not always the case, since an item may be perfectly valid in logical and theoretical terms, yet remain a non-predictor of health care behaviour due (eg) to educational or other factors in a specific study context.

29. An instrument's RELIABILITY may be defined as its capacity to produce similar results on retest.

30. Course members will be expected to identify and describe ONE such method from (eg) inter-rater reliability; test-retest reliability; and split half reliability.

D   USING OBSERVATIONAL INSTRUMENTS

31. An OBSERVATIONAL PROTOCOL may be defined as a set or series of rules or instructions, setting out the precise method for carrying out the observations in a specific study.

32. Course members should be able to give a good general account of the structure, use and analytic properties of the documentary analytic checklist.

33. By this is meant course members' ability effectively to record an individual observation; and subsequently to analyse and codify it, using the documentary analytic checklist. By "effective" here is meant that, when checked by the tutor, the observation must clearly characterise the documentary item(s) examined.

34. This item refers to course members' ability to record a whole sequence of useful observations; and subsequently to analyse them and describe the results, using the documentary analytic checklist.

35. Here course members should be able to give a good general description of the structural properties of the ward observation sheet; and of its use for recording, and subsequent coding and analysis of observations.

36. This skill is demonstrated by the ability to use the ward observation sheet and associated ward observation schedule effectively to record a few ward observations.

37. This skill is demonstrated by the ability to carry out a sustained sequence of observations, using the ward observation sheet and its associated ward observation schedule; subsequently effectively coding and analysing the data thus obtained.

38. This skill is demonstrated during discussion of an observation sequence; in which the course member is able to identify (1) his or her longer-term preparations for the observational sessions; (2) more immediate preparations, carried out just prior to an observation session; (3) the protocol followed during the observation session itself; (4) data analysis coding and storage for subsequent retrieval following the observation session. This skill may additionally be checked by tutorial observation before, during and after observational sequences.

39. Here the course member must demonstrate effective strategies for data storage and retrieval , including (eg) use of files and/or ring binders; card indices; and/or transfer to electronic storage.

40. This skill is demonstrated by the course member's manifest ability to produce data codings, summaries and analyses; and to display these in the form of tallies, tables, pie/bar charts or histograms, and/or verbal summaries as required.

OBSERVATIONAL DATABASE FORMAT AND ANALYSIS

R3 Ward Observations:

```
┌─────────────────────────────────────────────────────────────────┐
│  Sheet and Obs No:  10.2      Date:  17.10.89      Day:  3        │
│                                                                   │
│  Time Code:  6              Staff Code:  13      Staff Grade:  NA │
│                                                                   │
│  Description:  Supervising patients showering and talking to patient │
│                                                                   │
│  Descripcode:  sp      Care Type:  2  PN Code:  n                 │
│                                                                   │
│  RTA Code:  a Language:  7          NV Code:  -----               │
│                                                                   │
│  Location:  br          S-P Ratio:  1-1                           │
├─────────────────────────────────────────────────────────────────┤
│  SHEET AND OBS NO:       Record No 7                              │
│                                                                   │
│  Data records:  2,855       Selected:  193                       │
└─────────────────────────────────────────────────────────────────┘
```

C:\MF\R3.MFL   General help = F1

Annexe J shows the observational database as seen on the computer VDU. In the top box are the fourteen data fields of the Ward Observation Schedule (see Annexe A). The data is transferred from each observation sheet and entered into the appropriate field of the database.

To analyse the data simple frequency counts are carried out, for example, to find out how many description codes relating to supervision of patients (sp) the following formula is inputted: descripcode (the field to which the code belongs) = sp.

The database then calculates out of the total number of observations how many relate to sp (supervision of patients). As can be seen in the bottom box there is a total of 2,855 data records and the analysis has selected 193 in relation to sp. Any combination of the data fields can be compared against each other and subsequently counted and given in the selected column. For key word searchers a simple command of *=(key word) is inputted and again subsequent frequencies and records are displayed.

The following table shows the frequency analysis for the non-nursing process and nursing process observation categories collected within the study. This was carried out by using string-scanning techniques within Masterfile PC database using the following example command, eg, the first line of the table AS (administrative supervisory) denotes how many times staff on R1 ward interacted within the administrative supervisory category. With the Maples file open the command would be description code = AS. This would then give the frequency at the bottom of the VDU in relation to R1 which is 185. The same applies for each data field, eg, the data field = the observation code. The same applies for counting the frequencies for each data field.

In order to carry out field comparisons the following commands are used (name of field)=field code| (name of field)=field code. Any number of field comparisons can be compared together providing they are relevant.

Frequency of observations within each care category

OBSERVATION CODES	FREQUENCY				
	R1	R2	R3	E2	E1
AS	185	743	613	445	748
SP	434	542	656	262	250
PF	412	83	198	223	298
PS	852	670	355	340	470
NP	516	545	498	497	371
MS	235	212	243	892	562
CE	273	170	137	184	216
DM	93	32	154	168	54
AI	27	15	39	16	3
AE	33	50	24	175	34
PI	8	8	1	0	23
PE	44	62	3	21	21

Frequency of observations within each care category continued

OBSERVATION CODES	FREQUENCY				
	R1	R2	R3	E2	E1
II	54	32	0	26	42
IE	268	246	208	40	151
EI	37	73	124	18	67
EE	43	59	83	143	29
INDIRECT	1513	1939	1870	2280	1885
GROUP	81	253	419	231	426
DIRECT	767	796	426	424	655

Observation trend analysis
600 through 3000 observations

The following table is a further example of frequency analysis for non-nursing process and nursing process observation categories. The table identifies the frequencies for each care category at intervals from 600 through 3000. The non-nursing observation codes were used for the basis of the analysis in Figure 5.

Frequency of observations within care categories from
600 through to 3000 observations

OBSERVATION CODES	600	1200	1800	2400	3000
AS	132	291	449	605	743
SP	124	201	305	379	542
PF	5	26	58	63	83
PS	141	313	421	521	670
NP	104	207	315	488	545

OBSERVATION CODES	600	1200	1800	2400	3000
MS	67	86	131	180	212
CE	16	56	97	140	170
DM	11	21	22	27	32
AI	13	13	15	15	15
AE	9	33	34	50	50
PI	-	1	1	8	8
PE	4	27	38	58	62
II	-	-	10	32	32
IE	60	70	131	206	246
EI	7	36	52	62	73
EE	11	27	34	57	59
INDIRECT	427	852	1214	1583	1939
GROUP	40	61	159	199	253
DIRECT	129	280	413	609	796

Qualitative analysis

String-scanning techniques were used for qualitative analysis to support the quantitative data. In order to examine the range of behaviours of charge nurses in relation to their administration role the following commands were used to access relevant data (description code)=as (staff grade)=cn. The VDU then displays all the relevant data records relating to the charge nurse and administration. By using a special screen format all the "time capsules" or descriptions can be grouped together for further analysis.

By using this type of analysis it is possible to page through the descriptions of care and pull out the relevant qualitative detail to describe the nature of activities that the charge nurse (cn) undertook in the administrative (as) role. The following are a partial print out of the database descriptions in relation to the above criteria and were used for the basis of partial analysis identified in the observational findings.

String scanning for qualitative detail

OBSERVATION CODE	DESCRIPTION
as	Writing daily report sheet
as	Writing daily report sheet
as	Writing daily report sheet
as	Writing daily report sheet
as	Writing day report sheet
as	Writing day report sheet
as	Talking to sn visiting ward
as	Talking to sn visiting ward
as	Writing in diary
as	In conversation with nurse about duty times
as	Answering question from a nurse visiting the ward
as	Talking to staff nurse about article he will order for the ward
as	Writing in nurses notes of patient file
as	Writing in nurses notes of patient file
as	Talking to snm about staff levels
as	Sorting through paperwork on desk. Signing letter.

CENTRAL NOTTINGHAMSHIRE HEALTH AUTHORITY
PSYCHIATRIC NURSING AUDIT WARD E1

Grade	All staffs
Number of W. T. E	18.80
Total number of hours observed	145.17
Morning period	
% time spent in direct care (individual)	13.78
% time spent in direct care (group)	30.45
% time spent in indirect care	16.03
% time spent in associated work	26.60
% time spent in personal work	13.14
Afternoon period	
% time spent in direct care (individual)	3.72
% time spent in direct care (group)	23.50
% time spent in indirect care	34.96
% time spent in associated work	36.68
% time spent in personal work	1.15
Evening period	
% time spent in direct care (individual)	6.19
% time spent in direct care (group)	45.71
% time spent in indirect care	21.43
% time spent in associated work	11.43
% time spent in personal work	15.24
Overall	
% time spent in direct care (individual)	7.92
% time spent in direct care (group)	31.34
% time spent in indirect care	24.91
% time spent in associated work	26.98
% time spent in personal work	8.84

COMPARISON DATA

DIRECT CARE/GROUP WORK	7.92	INDIRECT CARE	24.91
	31.34		26.98
	39.26		8.84
			60.73

G1 UNIVERSITY HOSPITAL TRUST - QUALITY DEPARTMENT

Report 9   CARE TYPE BY GRADE OF STAFF (Percentage)

Indirect Care: No interaction between nurse and patient took place (but, for example, care could have been planned).

Direct Care: Interaction between nurse and patient took place on a one-to-one basis

Staff	Total	Percentage of Care Type	
		Indirect Care	Direct Care
Grade A	100	71.00	29.00
Grade B	243	79.84	20.16
Grade E	66	92.42	7.58
Grade G	20	95.00	5.00
Student	372	57.26	42.74
Totals	801	65.00	35.00

G2 UNIVERSITY TRUST HOSPITAL

EARLY   DAY 1   WARD 3A
DATE: 19-10-92

TOTAL TIME IN MINUTES

DIRECT CARE	180
INDIRECT CARE	75
SUPPORT	
HOUSEKEEPING	70
ADMINISTRATION	5
EDUCATION	100
OTHER	50
TOTAL TIME	480
DIRECT CARE %	37%
INDIRECT CARE %	63%

R5 WARD - SEPTEMBER 1993

Report 9   CARE TYPE BY GRADE OF STAFF (Percentage)

Indirect Care: No interaction between nurse and patient took place (but, for example, care could have been planned).

Group Care: Interaction between more than one nurse and/or more than one patient took place.

Direct Care: Interaction between nurse and patient took place on a one-to-one basis.

Staff	Total	Percentage		
		Indirect Care	Group Care	Direct Care
Grade B	348	54.89	4.31	40.80
Grade D	92	66.30	1.09	32.61
Grade E	256	64.45	1.17	34.38
Team Leader	128	74.22	0.78	25.00
Ward Manager	92	91.30	0.00	8.70
Totals	916	65.07	2.18	32.75

Report 9   CARE TYPE BY GRADE OF STAFF (Percentage)

Indirect Care: No interaction between nurse and patient took place (but, for example, care could have been planned).

Group Care: Interaction between more than one nurse and/or more than one patient took place.

Direct Care: Interaction between nurse and patient took place on a one-to-one basis.

R6 WARD BASE LINE MEASURE - JUNE 1993

Staff	Total	Percentage		
		Indirect Care	Group Care	Direct Care
Grade B	1158	63.47	1.99	34.54
Grade D	590	64.75	1.53	33.73
Grade E	507	76.33	0.20	23.47
Team Leader	197	87.82	0.00	12.18
Student	12	100.00	0.00	0.00
Ward Manager	36	100.00	0.00	0.00
Totals	2500	69.00	1.32	29.68

R6 WARD RE-MEASURE - DECEMBER 1993

Staff	Total	Percentage		
		Indirect Care	Group Care	Direct Care
Grade B	434	57.37	1.15	41.47
Grade D	135	60.74	4.44	34.81
Grade E	233	75.54	3.00	21.46
Student	16	100.00	0.00	0.00
Ward Manager	32	100.00	0.00	0.00
Totals	850	65.29	2.12	32.59

R4 WARD BASELINE AND REMEASURE

Report 9   CARE TYPE BY GRADE OF STAFF (Percentage)

Indirect Care:	No interaction between nurse and patient took place (but, for example, care could have been planned).
Group Care:	Interaction between more than one nurse and/or more than one patient took place.
Direct Care:	Interaction between nurse and patient took place on a one-to-one basis.

R4 BASE LINE MEASURE - DECEMBER 1992

		Percentage		
Staff	Total	Indirect Care	Group Care	Direct Care
Grade B	735	55.24	3.67	41.09
Grade D	465	61.94	3.01	35.05
Grade E	841	57.19	3.69	39.12
Team Leader	400	64.75	2.50	32.75
Student	72	75.00	11.11	13.89
Ward Manager	85	84.71	1.18	14.12
Totals	2598	60.05	3.50	36.45

R4 WARD RE-MEASURE - FEBRUARY 1994

		Percentage		
Staff	Total	Indirect Care	Group Care	Direct Care
Grade B	703	47.23	8.39	44.38
Grade D	257	43.58	7.39	49.03
Grade E	854	50.82	6.56	42.62
Team Leader	299	65.89	3.34	30.77
Student	251	71.71	19.92	8.37
Totals	2364	53.09	8.21	38.71

References

Aggleton, P and Chalmers, H (1986): 'Nursing Research, Nursing Theory and the Nursing Process'. *Journal of Advanced Nursing*, Vol 11, No 2, pp 197-202.

Akinsanya, J A (1984): 'The Use of Theories in Nursing. *Nursing Times*, Vol 80, No 14, pp 59-60.

Akinsanya, J A (1985): 'A Slow Process'. *Nursing Times*, Vol 81, No 43, pp 25-27.

Akinsanya, J A (1986): 'Poorly Prepared'. *Senior Nurse,* Vol 4, No 6, pp 32-33.

Akinsanya, J A (1986a): 'Science at Work'. *Senior Nurse*, Vol 4, No 4, pp 28-30.

Akinsanya, J A (1988): Making Research Useful to the Nurse Practitioner. Paper presented at the Inaugural Research Conference: Foundations of Nursing Research. Rampton Hospital, June, 1988.

Alexander, M F (1980): *Nurse Education: An Experiment in Integration of Theory and Practice in Nursing*. Unpublished Phd thesis. University of Edinburgh.

Alexander, M F (1983): *Learning to Nurse*. Edinburgh: Churchill Livingstone.

Ashworth, P (1985): *How Much Change?* Manchester, University of Manchester.

Baines, L (1981): 'Fully Involved'. *Nursing Times,* Vol 77, No 29, pp 1262-1264.

Baker, C, West J, Stern P (1992): 'Method Slurring: The Grounded Theory/ Phenomenological Examples'. *Journal of Advanced Nursing*, Vol 17, No 11, pp 1356-1358.

Baker, R (1993): 'Avedis Donabedian: An Interview'. *Quality in Health Care,* Vol 2, No 2, pp 40-46.

Ball, J A, Goldstone, L A, Collier, M M (1984): Criteria for Care: The Manual of the North West Nurse Staffing Levels Project. Newcastle upon Tyne Products Ltd.

Balogh, R (1991): Psychiatric Nursing Audit: A Study of Practice: Garlands Hospital.

Barnett, D, Wainwright, P (1987): 'A Measure of Quality'. *Senior Nurse,* Vol 6, No 3, pp 8-9.

Barnett, D, Wainwright, P (1987a): 'Between Two Tools'. *Senior Nurse,* Vol 6, No 4, pp 40-41.

Barnett, D, Wainwright, P (1987b): 'The Right Reflection'. *Senior Nurse,* Vol 6, No 5, pp 33-36.

Barrowclough, C, Whitmore, B, Tessier, I (1984): 'The Same Only Different'. *Nursing Mirror,* Vol 159, No 15, pp 28-30.

Bowman, G S, Parsons, C M, Pointon, W (1983): 'The Pitfalls of Implementing the Nursing Process'. *Nursing Times,* Vol 79, No 2, pp 29-35.

Bradshaw, S (1987): 'Phaneuf's Nursing Audit'. In Pearson, A (ed): *Nursing Quality Measurement.* Chichester: John Wiley and Sons.

Brenner, M (1985): 'Intensive Interviewing'. In Brenner, M, Brown, J, Canter, D (eds) (1985): *The Research Interview, Uses and Approaches,* pp 147-162. London: Academic Press.

Brooking, J I (1986): *Patient and Family Participation in Nursing Care: The Development of a Nursing Process Measurement Scale.* Kings College, University of London: unpublished PhD thesis.

Brooking, J I (1988): 'A Scale to Measure Use of the Nursing Process'. *Nursing Times,* April 12th, Vol 85, No 15, pp 44-48.

Brittle, J, Marsh, J (1986): 'Monitor: Definition or Measurement? *Nursing Times,* Vol 82, No 45, pp 36-37.

Bryant, J H (1975): 'Health Care Trends and Nursing Roles'. In Leininger, M (1975): *Barriers and Facilitators to Quality Health Care: Health Care Dimensions.* Philadelphia: F A Davies and Co.

Burrow, S (1992): 'The Deliberate Self-Harming Behaviour of Patients within a British Special Hospital'. *Journal of Advanced Nursing,* Vol 17, No 2, pp 138-148.

Butterworth, T (1994): *Working in Partnership: A Collaborative Approach to Care. Report of the Mental Health Nursing Review Team.* Department of Health. London: HMSO.

Carter, M A (1985): 'The Philosophical Dimensions of Qualitative Nursing Science Research'. In Leininger, M (1985): *Qualitative Research Methods in Nursing.* London: Grune and Stratton.

Carton, G, Langton, D, Robinson, D K (1990): 'Teaching the Nursing Process'. *Nursing Standard,* Vol 5, No 8, pp 23-27.

Carton, G (1994): *Effects of a Customised Teaching Package on Nursing Process in a Special Hospital.* Anglia Polytechnic University: unpublished diploma dissertation.

Collins, M (1990): *How Grade Affects the Activities of Nurses with Regard to Nursing Care. Rampton Hospital.* Unpublished diploma dissertation.

Cormack, D F S (1976): *Psychiatric Nursing Observed.* London: Royal College of Nursing.

Cormack, D F S (1983): *Psychiatric Nursing Described.* New York: Churchill Livingstone.

Cowman, S (1993): 'Triangulation: A Means of Reconciliation in Nursing Research'. *Journal of Advanced Nursing,* Vol 18, No 5, pp 788-792.

Curl, M, Robinson, D K, Reed, V (1993): *The Use of Hand-held Computers in Clinical Observational Audit.* Department of Health/Rampton Hospital.

Curtis, B J (1985): 'Auditing: A Method for Evaluating Quality of Care'. *JONA,* Vol 15, No 10, pp 24-26.

Davis, B D (1984): 'Interviews with Student Nurses about their Training'. *Nurse Education Today,* Vol 4, No 6, pp 136-140.

Davis, B D (1981): 'Social Skills in Nursing'. In Argyle, M (ed): *Social Skills and Health.* London: Methuen.

Davis, B D (1983): 'Students' Perceptions of their Significant Others' (p48). In Davis, B D (ed): 1983: *Research into Nurse Education.* London: Croom Helm.

Davis, B D (1986a): 'A Review of Recent Psychiatric Research in Psychiatric Nursing. In Brooking, J ed: *Psychiatric Nursing Research,* pp 3-19. Chichester: John Wiley and Sons.

Davis, B D (1986b): 'Culture and Psychiatric Nursing: Implications for Training'. In Cox, J L (ed): *Transcultural Psychiatry,* pp 218-233. Beckenham: Croom Helm.

Davies, M Z (1986c): 'Observation in Natural Settings'. In Chenitz, W C, Swanson, J M (eds): *From Practice to Grounded Theory: Qualitative Research in Nursing,* pp 48-65. Menlo Park: CA: Addison-Wesley Publishing Company.

De La Cuesta, C (1983): 'The Nursing Process from Development to Implementation. *Journal of Advanced Nursing,* Vol 8, No 5, pp 365-371.

Denzin, N (1970): 'Strategies of Multiple Triangulation'. In *The Research Act,* pp 297-311. New York, McGraw Hill.

Dickson, N (1987): 'Do you Measure Up?' *Nursing Times,* November, Vol 83, No 44, pp 26-28.

Department of Health (1988): *Service Quality Study*, p 17. London: Department of Health.

Department of Health (1989a): *Working for Patients*. London: HMSO.

Department of Health (1989b): *A Strategy for Nursing (1). Report of the Steering Committee*. London: Department of Health.

Department of Health (1989c): *Caring for People: Community Care in the Next Decade and Beyond*. London: HMSO.

Department of Health (1991): *The Patients' Charter*. London: HMSO.

Department of Health (1992): *The Health of the Nation: A Strategy for Health in England*. London: HMSO.

Department of Health (1993a): *A Strategy for Nursing, Midwifery and Health Visiting Research (2)*. London: Department of Health.

Department of Health (1993b): *A Vision for the Future*. London: National Health Service Management Executive, April 1993.

Donabedian, A (1966): *The Definition of Quality Assessment and Monitoring*. Michigan: Health Administration Press.

Donabedian, A (1993): 'Avedis Donabedian: An Interview by Richard Baker'. *Quality in Health Care*, Vol 2, No 2, pp 40-46.

Draper, J (1992): 'The Impact of Nursing Models'. *Senior Nurse*, Vol 12, No 3, pp 38-39.

Dukes, J and Stewart, R (1993): 'Be Prepared'. *Health Service Journal*, Vol 103, No 5337, pp 24-25.

Ellis, M (1987): 'Quality: Who Cares?' *British Journal of Occupational Therapy*, Vol 50, No 6, pp 195-200.

Ellis, R (ed) (1988): *Professional Competence and Quality Assurance in the Caring Professions*. Croom Helm.

Field, P A, Morse, J M (1985): *Nursing Research: The Application of Qualitative Approaches*. Chatham: Mackay.

Flowers, H H (1982): 'Some Simple Apple II Software for the Collection and Analysis of Observational Data'. *Behaviours Research Methods and Instrumentation*, Vol 14, No 2, pp 241-9.

Glaser, B G, Strauss, A C (1967): *The Discovery of Grounded Theory: Strategies for Qualitative Research*. New York: Aldine Publishing Company.

Goldstone, L (1987): In Pearson, A (ed): *Nursing Quality Measurement*. Chichester: John Wiley and Sons, Chapter 5, pp 53-59.

Goldstone, L, Ball, J, Collier, M (1983): *Monitor*. Newcastle upon Tyne: Polytechnic Publications.

Gould, E J (1985): 'Standardised Home Health Nursing Care Plans: A Quality Assurance Tool. *Quality Review Bulletin*, Vol 11, No 11, pp 334-348.

Green, R (1987): 'Measures of Quality in Mental Health'. *Hospitals and Health Services Review*, September 1987, pp 215-218.

Green, W, Hinchcliff, S, Fordham, J, Schober, J (1991): *Quality Assurance.* Distance Learning Centre, South Bank Polytechnic.

Greenhalgh and Company Limited (1992): *Observational Data Capture through the Use of Hand-held Devices.* GCL Activity Analysis, GCL House, Macclesfield, Cheshire, SK11 7JL.

Harrison, D N (1994): *Audit for Nursing Services. Nursing Services for Prisoners.* London: HM Prison Service Health Care.

Hardy, L, Engel, J (1987): 'The Search for Professionalism'. *Nursing Times*, Vol 83, No 15, pp 37-39.

Harre, R, Secord, P F (1972): *The Explanation of Social Behaviour.* Oxford: Basil Blackwell.

Hayward, J C (1986): *Report of the Nursing Process Evaluation Working Group.* London: Kings College, University of London.

Henderson, V (1982): 'The Nursing Process: Is the Title Right?'. *Journal of Advanced Nursing*, Vol 7, No 2, pp 103-109.

Hegyvary, S T, Haussman, P K D (1976): 'Monitoring Nursing Care Quality'. *Journal of Nursing Administration,* Vol 6, No 9, pp 3-9.

Hilton, J, Dawson, J (1988): 'Monitor Evaluated'. *Senior Nurse,* Vol 8, No 9, pp 3-9.

Hilton, I, Dawson, J (1988a): 'Monitor and Criteria for Care: The Portsmouth Experience'. *Senior Nurse*, Vol 8, No 6, pp 26-28.

Hughes, C P (1991): 'Community Psychiatric Nursing and the Depressed Elderly: A Case for using Cognitive Therapy'. *Journal of Advanced Nursing*, Vol 16, No 5, pp 565-572.

Hume, D (1739): *A Treatise of Human Nature,* Book I, Part III, Section xiv; Book III, Part I, Section i. Many editions; but see that edited by D G C Macnabb, Glasgow, Fontana/Collins, 1978.

Hunt, J (1985): *Nursing Care Plans: The Nursing Process at Work.* New York: John Wiley and Sons.

Hunt, J (1987): 'Assuring Quality'. *Nursing Times*, Vol 83, No 44, pp 29-31.

Hunt, J (1990): *Quality Assurance and Nursing.* London: King's Fund Centre.

Hurst, K (1990): *Analysing Psychiatric Nursing Care.* Central Notts Health Authority: Paper prepared for internal circulation.

Hurst, K, Dean, A (1987): 'An Investigation into Nurses' Perceptions of Problem-Solving in Clinical Practice'. In Hannah, K J, Reimer, M et al; *Clinical Judgement and Decision Making: The Future with Nursing Diagnosis*, pp 409-411. New York: John Wiley and Sons.

Hurst, K, Howard, D (1988): 'Measure for Measure'. *Nursing Times,* June, Vol 84, No 22, pp 30-32.

Hurst, K, Howard, D (1989): *Psychiatric Audit Results,* Millbrook Mental Health Unit, Mansfield.

Hurst, K (1992): 'Changes in Nursing Practice 1884-1992'. *Nursing Times,* Vol 88, No 22, pp 30-32.

Hurst, K, Quinn, H (1992): *Nursing Establishment and Skill Mix in Northern Ireland. Making the Best Use of Nursing Resources in the Province,* pp 21-23. Nuffield Institute and Northern Ireland Office, Leeds.

Hurst, K (1993): *Nursing Workforce Planning,* p 74. Harlow: Longman.

Jones, P (1979): 'A Terminology for Nursing Diagnoses'. *Advances in Nursing Science,* October 1979, p 69.

Kirwin, B (1980): 'Nursing Process: From the Ivory Tower to the Ward Floor'. *Nursing Mirror,* Vol 150, No 9, pp 36-38.

King, R D, Raynes, N V, Tizard, J (1971): *Patterns of Residential Care: Sociological Studies in Institutions for Handicapped Children.* London: Routledge and Kegan Paul.

Kitson, A (1986): 'Indicators in Quality in Nursing Care: An Alternative Approach'. *Journal of Advanced Nursing,* Vol 11, No 2, pp 133-134.

Kitson, A (1990): *Quality Patient Care: The Dynamic Standard Setting System.* RCN Standards of Care Project, Middlesex: Scutari Projects.

Kitson, A (1990): *The Dynamic Standard Setting System.* London: Scutari Projects.

Kleinman, A, Good, B (1985): 'Depression and the Culture Bound Syndrome; In Kleinman, A, Good, B, eds (1985): *Culture and Depression.* Berkley: University of California Press.

Kleinman, A (1987): 'Anthropology and Psychiatry: The Role of Culture in Cross-Cultural Research in Illness. *British Journal of Psychiatry,* Vol 151, pp 447-454.

Lambersten, E C (1965): 'Evaluating the Quality of Nursing Care'. *Hospitals J.A.H.A.,* Vol 39, pp 61-62.

Lamonica, E L (1979): *The Nursing Process: A Humanistic Approach.* New York: Addison-Wesley.

Lawler, J (1991): 'In Search of an Australian Identity'. In *Towards a Discipline of Nursing* (Gray, G and Pratt, R eds). Melbourne: Churchill Livingstone, p 217.

Lechl, A, Kuderling, I, Kurre, I and Fuchs, E (1988): 'Locomotor activity registration by passive infrared detection in saddle back tamarins and tree shrews. *Physiology and Behaviour,* Vol 4, No 2, pp 281-4.

Leddy, S and Pepper, J M (1993): *Conceptual Basis of Professional Nursing, 3rd Edition.* Philadelphia, J B Lippincott, p 293.

Leininger, M (1975): 'Health Care Systems for Tomorrow: Possibilities and Guidelines'. In Leininger, M ed (1975): *Barriers and Facilitators to Quality Health Care: Health Care Dimensions.* Philadelphia: F A Davies Company.

Leininger, M (1978): *Transcultural Nursing: Concepts, Theories and Practices.* New York: John Wiley and Sons.

Leininger, M (1979): *Transcultural Nursing.* New York: Masson Publications.

Leininger, M (1981): *Caring: An Essential Human Need* (Proceedings of the Three National Caring Conferences). Thoroughfare, N J: Charles B Slack Inc.

Leininger, M (1984): 'Transcultural Nursing: An Essential Knowledge and Practice Field for Today'. *The Canadian Nurse,* December 1984, Vol 80, No 11, pp 41-45.

Leininger, M (1985): 'Ethnography and Ethnonursing: Models and Modes of Qualitative Data Analysis'. In Leininger, M ed: *Qualitative Research Methods in Nursing.* Orlando: Grune and Stratton.

Leininger, M (1986): 'Care Facilitation and Resistance factors in the Changing Culture of Nursing'. *TOP-Clinical Nurse,* Vol 8, No 2, pp 1-12.

Leininger, M (1987): 'Importance and Uses of Ethnomethods: Ethnography and Ethnonursing Research'. In Cahoon, M ed: *Recent Advances in Nursing.* London: Churchill Livingstone.

Leininger, M (1990): 'A New and Changing Decade Ahead: Are Nurses Prepared?' *Journal of Transcultural Nursing,* Vol 1, No 2, p1 (editorial).

Leininger, M (1992): 'Current Issues, Problems and Trends to Advance Qualitative Paradigmatic Research Methods for the Future. *Qualitative Health Research,* Vol 2, No 4, pp 392-415.

Lesnik, M, Anderson, B (1955): *Nursing Practice and the Law* (second edition). Philadelphia: Lippincott.

Lewis, M H, Baumeister, A A and McCorkie, D L (1985): 'A Computer Supported Method for Analysing Behavioural Observations: Studies with Stereotypy. *Psychopharmacology,* Vol 85, No 2, pp 204-209.

Lian, W A (1985): 'How do we give Quality Care in this Age of Modern Technology?' *Nursing Journal of Singapore,* 24 June, pp 21-26.

Liddle, B, Gilby, S (1991): 'Personalising the Service: Quality in Action'. *International Journal of Health Care Quality Assurance,* Vol 4, No 2, pp 4-8.

Lincoln, Y, Guba, G (1985): *Naturalistic Inquiry.* Beverley Hills, CA: Sage.

Lorentzon, M (1987): 'Quality in Nursing: The State of the Art'. *Senior Nurse,* Vol 7, No 6, pp 11-12.

Lynch-Sauer, J (1985): 'Using Phenomenological Research Methods to Study Nursing Phenomena. In Leininger, M ed: *Qualitative Research Methods in Nursing*. London: Grune and Stratton.

Mackie, L C R, Welch, J W (1982): 'Quality Assurance Audit for the Nursing Process. *Nursing Times*, Vol 78, No 42, pp 1757-1758.

Marriner, A (1986): *Nursing Theorists and their Work*. Saint Louis: The C V Mosby Company.

Mayers, M G (1986): *A Systematic Approach to the Nursing Care Plan*. New York: Prentice-Hall inc.

Mental Health Act (1983): *Draft Code of Practice*. London: HMSO.

McCaugherty, D (1990): *The Integration of Theory and Practice in Student Nurses*. University of Bath: Unpublished PhD thesis.

McCaugherty, D (1992a): 'Integrating Theory and Practice'. *Senior Nurse*, Vol 12, No 1, pp 36-37.

McCaugherty, D (1992b): 'The Gap Between Nursing Theory and Practice'. *Senior Nurse*, Vol 12, No 6, pp 44-48.

McFarland, G et al (1990): 'Knowledge about Care and Caring. Group IV: Behaviour Problems/Mental Illness: Addictions. *ANA American Academic Nurse*, G-177, pp 135-139.

Meichenbaum, D H (1977): *Cognitive Behaviour Modification*. New York: Plenum.

Mill, J S (1840: 'A System of Logic'. Quoted in Passmore, J (1970), *A Hundred Years of Philosophy* (John Stuart Mill and British Empiricism), pp 13-34. Harmondsworth, Penguin Books.

Milne, D, Turton, N (1986): 'Making the Nursing Process Work in Mental Health'. *Senior Nurse*, Vol 5, No 5/6, pp 33-36.

Mitchell, T (1984): 'The Nursing Process Debate: Is Nursing Any Business of Doctors?' *Nursing Times*, Vol 80, No 19, pp 28-32.

Moores, E (1993): *Preface to "A Vision for the Future"*, Department of Health. London: National Health Service Management Executive, April 1993.

Moores, B, Grant, G W B (1976): 'On the Nature and Incidence of Staff-Patient Interactions in Hospitals for the Mentally Handicapped'. *International Journal of Nursing Studies*, Vol 13, pp 69-81.

Moores, B, Moult, A (1979): 'Patterns of Nurse Activity'. *Journal of Advanced Nursing*, Vol 4, No 2, pp 137-149.

Mulligan, B (1972): 'How Many Nurses Equal Enough'. *Nursing Times*, April 13, pp 428-430.

Mulligan, B (1973): *Measurement of Patient-Nurse Dependency and Workload Indices*. London: King's Fund Project Paper.

National Health Service Act (1977): London: HMSO.

Neisser, U (1976): *Cognition and Reality*, pp 1, 9, 50. San Francisco, W H Freeman.

Newman, M (1979): *Theory Development in Nursing*. Philadelphia: F A Davies Company.

Nicholas, B (1969): 'Do Mental Nurse Have a Future? Report on a Conference'. *Nursing Times*, Vol 65, No 40, pp 1272-73.

Norman, J (1991): *An Investigation into the Education of Theatre Nursing Prior to the Implementation of the Nursing Process*. Lincoln County Hospital/Rampton Hospital: Unpublished diploma thesis.

Nursing Times (1990): 'Editorial: Lets Face it'. *Nursing Times*, Vol 76, No 43, p 1859.

Oliver, S (1991): 'Quality Care'. *Nursing Standard Supplement*, October, Vol 6, No 2, p 4.

Openshaw, S (1984): 'Literature Review': Measurement of Adequate Care'. *International Journal of Nursing Studies*, Vol 21, No 4, pp 295-304.

Ovretveit, P (1990): 'What is Quality in Health Services?' *Health Services Management*, Vol 86, No 3, pp 132-133.

Owens, M (1989): *Psychiatric Nursing Audit*. Results for Trent Ward, August 1989, Millbrook Mental Health Unit, Sutton Ashfield.

Pearson, A (1986): *Introducing New Norms in a Nursing Unit and Analysis of the Process of Change*. University of London: Unpublished PhD thesis.

Peplau, H E (1994): 'Psychiatric Mental Health Nursing: Challenge and Change'. *Journal of Psychiatric and Mental Health Nursing*, Vol 1, No 1, pp 3-7.

Phaneuf, M (1976): *The Nursing Audit*. New York: Appleton-Century-Crofts.
Polit, D, Hungler, B (1989): *Essentials of Nursing Research*, pp 236-237. Philadelphia: J B Lippincott.

Powney, J, Watts, M (1987): *Interviewing in Educational Research*. London: Routledge and Kegan Paul.

Pringle, M (1992): 'From Theory to Practice in General Practice Audit'. *Quality in Health Care*, Vol 1, supplement, pp 12-14.

Proctor, S J (1993): 'Why Clinical Research Needs Medical Audit'. *Quality in Health Care*, Vol 2, No 1, pp 1-2.

Rafferty, D (1992): 'Implications of the Theory-Practice Gap for Project 2000 Students'. *British Journal of Nursing*, Vol 1, No 10, pp 507-513.

Reason, P (ed) (1989): *Human Inquiry in Action: Developments in New Paradigm Research*. Newbury Park, CA: Sage.

Redfern, S J, Norman, I J (1990): 'Measuring the Quality of Nursing Care: A Consideration of Alternative Approaches'. *Journal of Advanced Nursing*, Vol 15, No 11, pp 1260-1271.

Reinhartz, S (1983): *'Phenomenology as a Dynamic Process: Phenomenology and Pedagogy'*, Vol 1, pp 77-79.

Riehl, J, Roy, C (1980): *Conceptual Models for Nursing Practice* (Second Edition). New York: McGraw-Hill.

Reed, J (1993): 'Individualised Nursing Care: Some Implications'. *Journal of Clinical Nursing*, Vol 1, pp 7-12.

Reed, V (1978): *Analysing Ward Input for Handicapped Children*. Department of Psychology, University of Nottingham: unpublished PhD thesis.

Reed, V and Robinson, D K (1993): *The Rampton Hospital Community Nursing Liaison Service: Achievements and Opportunities*. Rampton Hospital.

Reed, V and Dean, A (1990): *The Bath and Mersey Projects: Professional Evaluation* - Two Detailed Interim Papers. London, Department of Health (Information Technology Branch).

Reed, V, Robinson, D K (1988): *Curricular Implications of Individualised Care in Forensic Nursing*. Paper given at the Sixth Annual Research in Education Conference, San Francisco, USA, January 1988.

Rhys-Hearn, C (1976): *Nursing Needs, Nursing Workload and Nursing Resources*. Proceedings of the Symposium on Medical Data Processing, Toulouse.

Rhys-Hearn, C, Potts, D (1977): 'The Effects of Patients' Individual Characteristics Upon Activity Items of Nursing Care'. *International Journal of Nursing Studies*, Vol 15, No 1, pp 23-30.

Rhys-Hearn, C (1979): 'Comparison of Rhys-Hearn Method of Determining Nursing Staff Requirements with the Aberdeen Formula'. *International Journal of Nursing Studies*, Vol 16, No 1, pp 95-103.

Rhys-Hearn, C (1979a): 'Staffing Geriatric Wards. Trials of a Package'. *Nursing Times Occasional Papers*, Vol 75, No 11, pp 45-48.

Robinson, D K (1987): *Rampton Hospital Nursing Process Study: A Report of a Pilot of the Ward Interaction Observation Schedule*. Rampton Hospital/Wakefield Health Authority.

Robinson, D K (1988): *Measuring Quality Care in a Special Hospital: An Approach through the Nursing Process*. Bournemouth University: unpublished diploma dissertation.

Robinson, D K (1988a): *Evaluative Study of the Nursing Process in a Special Hospital: A Process for Care*. Paper given at the First Annual Research Conference, Mersey Region Nursing Research Interest Group, March 1988.

Robinson, D K, Reed, V (1989): *Practitioner Research in Action*. Paper given at the Seventh Annual Research in Education Conference, San Francisco, USA, January 1989.

Robinson, D K (1989a): *Measuring Quality Care in a Special Hospital: An Approach through the Nursing Process.* Paper given at the multidisciplinary Research Interest Group, Rampton Hospital, Retford, Notts, March 1989.

Robinson, D K (1989b): *Measuring Quality Care: A Developing Qualitative Approach.* Paper given at the National Association for Quality Assurance, Malvern, November 1989.

Robinson, D K (1990): 'Two Decades of the Process' *Senior Nurse,* Vol 10, No 2, pp 4-6.

Robinson, D K (1990a): 'Qualitative Analysis of Quality Care'. *Senior Nurse,* Vol 10, No 7, pp 21-25.

Robinson, D K (1990b): *Observational Standards of Care Audit and Review.* Rampton Hospital.

Robinson, D K (1990c): *A Qualitative Approach to the Measurement of Quality Care.* Paper given at the International Quality Assurance Conference, Stockholm, Sweden, June 17-19, 1990.

Robinson, D K (1990d): *Measuring Quality Care: An Approach through the Nursing Process.* Paper given at the National Care Planning Group Conference, Kingsclere Centre, Basingstoke District Hospital, Berkshire, August 15, 1990.

Robinson, D K (1991): *Qualitative Measurement of the Process of Care.* Paper given at the First National QUAN Conference, Oxford University, July 1991.

Robinson, D K (1991a): *Developing Clinical Quality Indicators in Psychiatric Nursing.* Paper given at the Bournemouth University First National Quality Conference, September 1991.

Robinson, D K (1991b): *Developing Clinical Quality Indicators in Psychiatric Nursing.* Paper given at Loughborough University First National Quality Conference, September 1991.

Robinson, D K (1992): *The Advantages of Qualitative Approaches in the Measurement of Quality.* Paper given at the Psychiatric Nursing Audit Project, Newcastle University, May 1992.

Robinson, D K (1992a): *Documentary and Observational Audit Measures.* Paper given at the Health Sector of HM Prison Service, Home Office, London, September 1992.

Robinson, D K (1993): 'Hand-held Computers in Clinical Audit'. *Senior Nurse,* Vol 13, No 3, pp 14-17.

Robinson, D K (1993a): 'Computerised Observation Care Audit'. In *Managing Information for the Benefit of Patients.* Weybridge: BJHC Books.

Robinson, D K (1993b): 'Direct Downloading': A Route to Rapid Feedback. *Quality Connection,* July/August, Vol 2, Issue, 1, pp 1-2.

Robinson, D K (1993c): *The Use of Hand-held Computers for Data Capture in Clinical Audit.* Paper given at the National Quality Exhibition, Nottingham General Hospital, February 1993.

Robinson, D K (1993d): *Hand-held Computers in Observational Audit Data Collection.* Paper given at the Tenth Meeting, International Society for Quality Assurance, Maastricht, Netherlands, June 23, 1993.

Robinson, D K (1993e): *Hand-held Computers for Data Capture in Clinical Audit.* Paper given at the Third National Quality Assurance Conference, Heriot-Watt University, Edinburgh, July 20, 1993.

Robinson, D K (1993f): *Developing Clinical Quality Indicators in Psychiatric Nursing.* Paper given at the Institute of Psychiatry, November 1993.

Robinson, D K (1993g): *Computerised Observational Care Audit.* Paper given at the British Computer Society for Nursing Annual National Conference, Hinckley, November 1993.

Robinson, D K (1993h): *Research Data Collection and Analysis using Hand-held Computers.* Poster given at the Clinical Audit Conference, NEC, Birmingham, Department of Health, 1994.

Robinson, D K (1994): *Qualitative Measurement and Analysis of Care.* Royal College of Nursing Annual Nursing Research Conference, April 8-10, Grange Park Hotel, Hull.

Robinson, D K (1994a): *Developing Clinical Quality Indicators in Psychiatric Nursing.* Paper given at the Department of Health Vision for the Future Conference, Elephant and Castle, London, May 1994.

Rogers, M (1979): *An Introduction to the Theoretical Basis of Man.* Philadelphia: F A Davies Company.

Royal College of Nursing (1980): *Standards of Nursing Care.* London: RCN.

Royal College of Nursing (1981): *Towards Standards.* London: RCN.

Royal Liverpool University Trust Hospital (1992): *Staffing Activity Analysis, Ward 3A, Early Day 1* (19.10.92).

Roper, N, Logan, W, Tierney, A (1983): 'Is There a Danger of Processing Patients?' *Nursing Mirror,* Vol 156, No 2, pp 32-33.

Russell, B (1912): *The Problems of Philosophy.* London: Williams and Norgate.

Russell, B (1921): *The Analysis of Mind.* London: Allen and Unwin.

Sanbury, P R, Hagenmeyer, S H and Henault, M A (1985): 'Automated Measurement of Multivariate Locomotor Behaviour in Rodents. *Neurobehavioural Toxicology and Teratology,* Vol 7, No 1, pp 87-94.

Savage, P (1992): *Psychiatric Nurses' Attitudes Towards Nursing Process.* Bournemouth University: unpublished PhD thesis.

Schmadl, J C (1979): 'Quality Assurance: Examination of the Concept'. *Nursing Outlook,* Vol 27, No 7, pp 462-465.

Schmele, J A (1985): 'A Method for Evaluating Nursing Practice in a Community Setting'. *Quality Review Bulletin*, Vol 11, No 4, pp 115-122.

Shaw, C D (1986): *Introducing Quality Assurance*. London: King's Fund Centre.

Shaw, C (1988): 'Quality Assurance: A New Epidemic'. *NAHA News, June 1988, p1*.

Shaw, C (1989): *Medical Audit: A Hospital Handbook*. London: King's Fund Centre.

Shea, H L (1986): 'A Conceptual Framework to Study the Use of Nursing Care Plans. *International Journal of Nursing Studies*, Vol 23, No 2, pp 147-157.

Sheehan, J (1982): 'Educating Teachers: A Survey of the Opinion of Students'. *Journal of Advanced Nursing*, Vol 7, No 1, pp 69-77.

Sheehan, J (1986): 'Nursing Education in Britain: The State of the Art'. *Nurse Education Today*, Vol 6, No 1, pp 3-10.

Sheehan, J (1986a): 'Curriculum Models: Product Versus Process'. *Journal of Advanced Nursing*, vol 11, No 6, pp 671-678.

Sheehan, J (1989): *The Nature of the Nursing Process as a Concept in the Current Education of Nurses*. University of Leeds: unpublished PhD thesis.

Sheehan, J (1991): 'Conceptions of the Nursing Process Amongst Nurse Teachers and Clinical Nurses'. *Journal of Advanced Nursing*, Vol 16, No 3, pp 333-342.

Shotter, J (1981): 'Perception and Language: A Phenomenological Approach'. In Howarth, C I, Gillham, W E C eds: *The Structure of Psychology*, pp 667-683. London: George Allen and Unwin.

SHSA (1991): *Special Hospitals Service Authority Review: SHSA Explained.* London, SHSA.

Simpson, R B C (1989): 'Expressed Emotion and Nursing the Schizophrenic Patient. *Journal of Advanced Nursing*, Vol 14, No 6, pp 459-466.

Sines, D (1989): 'Meeting Consumer Needs: The Future Role of the Mental Handicap Nurse'. *The Professional Nurse*, September 1989, Vol 4, No 12, pp 593-597.

Sines, D (1989a): 'Towards Quality'. *Senior Nurse,* Vol 9, No 10, pp 9-11.

Smith, B (1986a): *The Nursing Process in Mental Handicap Nursing*. Kings College, University of London: dissertation submitted in partial fulfilment of requirements for BSc (Hons) Nursing Studies.

Smith, J P (1986): 'The Beginning of the End'. *Senior Nurse*, Vol 5, No 1, pp 14-15.

Smith, P (1986): *Research Methodology for Evaluating the Quality of Care: A Critique of Qualpacs Measuring Instrument.* Unpublished paper, RCN Research Society, 1986.

Stanton, A, Crotty, M (1991): 'The Impact of Research on Clinical Practice'. *Senior Nurse,* Vol 11, No 6, pp 16-18.

Stephenson, M (1984): 'Problems Remain'. *Nursing Mirror,* Vol 158, No 1 (supplement), pp v-vii.

Street, C G (1982): 'An Investigation of the Priority Placed on Nurse/Patient Interaction by Psychiatric Nurses'. In Brooking, J ed: *Psychiatric Nursing Research,* pp 26-29. Chichester, John Wiley and Sons.

Tanner, C (1987): 'Theoretical Perspectives for Research on Clinical Judgment'. In Hannah, K J, Reimer, M et al: *Clinical Judgement and Decision Making: The Future with Nursing Diagnosis,* pp 21-28. New York: John Wiley and Sons.

Tennant, I (1990): *Relationships between Planned and Delivered Care: An Observational Study.* Rampton Hospital: Unpublished diploma thesis.

Thompson, A (1979): 'The Nursing Process: Its Value for Special Hospital Patients'. *Nursing Mirror,* March, Vol 1, pp 20-21.

Tomalin, D (1991): *Auditing Quality Using Senior Monitor.* Paper given at First National Quality Assurance Network Conference, St Catherine's College, Oxford, July 1st.

Ventura, M R, Slakter, M J, Hageman, P T, Fox, R N (1989): 'Correlations of Two Quality of Nursing Care Measures'. *Nursing Management,* Vol 15, pp 507-513.

Wandelt, M A, Ager, J (1978): *Quality Patient Care Scale.* New York: Appleton-Century-Crofts.

Wandelt, M A, Stewart, D S (1975): *Slater Nursing Competency Rating Scale.* New York: Appleton-Century-Crofts.

Wainwright, P (1987): 'QUALPACS: a Practical Guide'. *The Professional Nurse,* October, Vol 3, No 1, pp 14-17.

Watson, J (1979): *The Philosophy and Science of Caring.* Boston: Little, Brown and Company.

West, B (1991): 'Auditing Quality'. *Nursing Standard Supplement,* October, Vol 2, No 2, p 5.

Whelan, J (1987): 'Using Monitor: Observer Bias'. *Senior Nurse,* Vol 7, No 6, pp 8-10.

White, A K (1993): 'The Nursing Process: A Constraint on Expert Practice'. *Journal of Nursing Management,* Vol 1, No 5, pp 542-252.

Whitfield, S (1989): 'Still Struggling with the Nursing Process'. *Nursing Standard,* Vol 3, No 23, pp 19-21.

Whitfield, M, Baker, R (1992): 'Measuring Patient Satisfaction for Audit in General Practice'. *Quality in Health Care*, Vol 1, No 3, pp 151-152.

Whyte, L, Youhill, G (1984): 'The Nursing Process in the Care of the Mentally Ill'. *Nursing Times*, Vol 80, No 5, pp 49-51.

Willard, C (1984): 'The Story of John'. *Nursing Mirror,* January 4, Vol 158, No 1, pp vii-viii.

Wilson-Barnett, J (1986): 'A Measure of Care'. *Nursing Times*, Vol 82, No 33, pp 57-58.

Wilson, G T (1980): 'Cognitive Factors in Lifestyle Changes: A Social Learning Perspective'. In Davidson, P O, Davidson, S M eds: *Behavioural Medicine: Changing Health Lifestyles,* pp 3-37, New York: Brunner-Mazel.